CLINICAL H

D0213330

CONTEMPORARY MATERNAL-NEWBORN NURSING CARE

FIFTH EDITION

Patricia Wieland Ladewig, PhD, RN
Professor and Academic Dean
School for Health Care Professions
Regis University
Denver, Colorado

Marcia L. London, MSN, RNC, NNP
Beth-El College of Nursing and Health Sciences
University of Colorado
Colorado Springs, Colorado

Sally B. Olds, MS, RNC, SANE
Professor Emerita
Beth-El College of Nursing and Health Sciences
Colorado Springs, Colorado

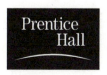

Prentice
Hall

Upper Saddle River, New Jersey 07458

Publisher: Julie Alexander
Executive Editor: Maura Connor
Editorial Assistant: Beth Ann Romph
Director of Manufacturing and Production: Bruce Johnson
Managing Editor: Patrick Walsh
Production Editor: Lisa Hessel, Carlisle Publishers Services
Production Liaison: Cathy O'Connell
Manufacturing Buyer: Pat Brown
Composition: Carlisle Communications, Ltd.
Printing and Binding: Banta Company

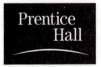

10 9 8 7 6 5 4 3 2 1
ISBN 0-13-032512-0

Preface

Your clinical experience this week will include one day at the local birthing center caring for three couplets (postpartum mother and her baby) and their families. On your other clinical day you will be making antepartal and postpartal home visits with a nurse in the home care department of the birthing center. As you begin your day in the birthing center, you are assigned to two couplets. One mother has just had her first baby by cesarean birth and is returning to her room. She has had epidural anesthesia and epidural morphine for postpartum pain control. Her baby is doing well and will be able to come to the mother's room for a visit as soon as the mother and father desire. The mother wants to begin breastfeeding as soon as possible. The second couplet is a 21-year-old gravida 1, para 1, mother who is also breastfeeding and will be going home with her baby after lunch. The mother and father are both deaf. You will be responsible for discharge teaching and arranging home visits. As a matter of fact, you will be present at the first home visit as part of your next clinical day.

As you organize your thoughts for today, think about your priorities. What special assessments and interventions will each mother and baby need? How will you assist the breastfeeding mothers? What different needs might you expect from the mother who has just had a cesarean and the mother who will soon be discharged? What additional assessments will be needed because of the postpartum epidural analgesia? How will you assist the deaf mother and father? Where will you find an interpreter? What resources are available in the community for both families?

The *Contemporary Maternal-Newborn Nursing Care Clinical Handbook* has been created to help you in situations just like these. The handbook provides succinct, pertinent information regarding the antepartum, intrapartum, newborn, and postpartum client. Each content area includes key information regarding medical therapy as well as nursing care information organized according to the nursing process. Critical nursing assessments and interventions are identified, and specific suggestions are given regarding documentation of care.

In addition to serving as a resource for normal and selected complications of childbearing, the handbook includes practical features to assist the nurse. Procedures specific to the maternal-child clinical area are included to help you provide nursing care. Commonly used medications are presented in the drug guide. A specially developed appendix with Spanish translations of some key phrases used in the maternal-child area will assist the nurse who does not speak Spanish. Another feature, Appendix I, contains information regarding working with deaf clients through an interpreter.

Although the handbook gives condensed information about each subject area, critical aspects of nursing practice have been presented. It is our hope that this book will enhance maternal-newborn nursing practice and help nurses provide safe, competent care to all mothers and babies.

We would like to express our appreciation to the Prentice-Hall team for their encouragement, support, and assistance. Three people in particular, merit special mention: Maura Connor, our editor, has been consistently enthusiastic, encouraging, and helpful throughout the process. We love working with her. Beth Romph, editorial assistant, supported us and responded to our needs with grace and good humor. And Lisa Hessel, the Production Coordinator at Carlisle Publisers Services, kept us on track with patience and unflappable calm.

Finally, we would like to express our heartfelt appreciation to our nursing students, who brighten each day. By being with them, we gained an understanding of their struggle to master an ever-growing body of knowledge. We have incorporated many of their requests and ideas into the information that appears in this handbook. As always, it is our goal to provide a tool that students and practicing nurses will find helpful.

PAL
MLL
SBO

Contents

PHOTOGRAPHIC CREDITS

CHAPTER 5
Figures 5–1, 5–2, and 5–9: © Elizabeth Elkin. Figures 5–5 and 5–6: Reprinted by permission of V. Dubowitz, M.D., Hammersmith Hospital, London, England.

CHAPTER 6
Figure 6–1: © Suzanne Arms Wimberley

CHAPTER 7
Figure 7–3: © Anne Dowie

CHAPTER 8
Figure 8–3: © Amy H. Snyder

ILLUSTRATORS

Kristin N. Mount, Nea Hanscomb, Joanne Bales/Precision Graphics, and George Kuper/Left Coast Group.

Chapter 1

The Antepartum Client

During the antepartal period, nursing interventions focus primarily on client teaching and ongoing monitoring of the woman so that any potential complications are detected promptly. Teaching typically focuses on nutrition, on interventions to deal with the common discomforts of pregnancy, and on self-care activities indicated throughout pregnancy.

Pregnancy Length

- Due date (date on which baby is expected) is calculated from the first day of a woman's last menstrual period (LMP). (See page 13 for description of calculation.)
- Pregnancy lasts about 9 calendar months, 10 lunar months, 40 weeks, or 280 days.
- Conception actually occurs about 14 days before the start of a woman's next menstrual period. Thus the actual time she is pregnant is about 2 weeks less, or 266 days.

Trimesters

- Pregnancy is discussed in terms of *trimesters,* which each last three calendar months.
- First trimester: The woman usually learns she is pregnant and may seek prenatal care. The first trimester is the time of primary organ development for the fetus.
- Second trimester: Considered the most tranquil for the pregnant woman. Morning sickness passes, and quickening (feeling the baby move) occurs.
- Third trimester: The woman becomes anxious for the pregnancy to end. She may feel awkward because of her increasing weight and the physical and psychologic changes she experiences.

Normal Physical Changes of Pregnancy

Uterus

- Dramatic increase in size and weight.
- **Braxton Hicks contractions** begin by the end of the first trimester. These are rhythmic contractions of the uterus that are painless initially but become noticeable, and sometimes uncomfortable, toward term (the end of pregnancy). They are then referred to as "false labor." Braxton Hicks contractions are palpable during bimanual exam by the 4th month and palpable abdominally by the 28th week.

Cervix

- Glandular tissue increases in number and becomes hyperactive.
- Mucous plug is formed in cervix and acts as a barrier to prevent ascending infection.
- Increased blood flow to cervix leads to softening (Goodell's sign) and bluish coloration (Chadwick's sign). Goodell's sign and Chadwick's sign are visible on speculum examination.

Ovaries

- Ovum production ceases.
- Corpus luteum persists and secretes hormones until weeks 10–12.

Vagina

- Increased vascularity produces bluish color (Chadwick's sign).
- Epithelium hypertrophies.

Breasts

- Increased size and nodularity; some increased tenderness.
- Superficial veins prominent.

- Increased pigmentation of areola and nipple.
- Colostrum is usually produced by week 12. (Colostrum is the antibody-rich forerunner of mature breast milk.) Women who are not visibly secreting colostrum need reassurance that they are producing it even if it is not evident.

Respiratory System

- Some hyperventilation occurs as pregnancy progresses.
- Increased tidal volume, decreased airway resistance.
- Diaphragm elevated, substernal angle increased.
- Breathing changes from abdominal to thoracic.

Cardiovascular System

- Blood volume increases about 45%.
- Decreased systemic and pulmonary vascular resistance.
- By weeks 24–28, cardiac output increases 30% to 50% over prepregnant levels; remains elevated for duration of pregnancy.
- Increased pulse rate.
- Blood pressure (BP) decreases slightly by second trimester; near prepregnant levels at term.
- Pressure of enlarging uterus on vena cava can interfere with blood return to the heart and cause dizziness, pallor, clamminess, and lowered BP. This condition is called *vena caval syndrome* or *supine hypotensive syndrome.* Research suggests that the uterus may also exert pressure on the aorta and its collateral circulation, making the term *aortocaval compression* more accurate (Wheeler, 1997). It is corrected by having the woman lie on her side or with a wedge under her right hip.
- Red blood cells (RBCs) and hemoglobin levels increase, as does the plasma level. Because plasma volume increases more, a **physiologic anemia of pregnancy** results, evident in an apparent decrease in hematocrit (Hct). Hct levels of 32% to 44% are considered normal.

- Leukocyte production increases to levels of $10,000-11,000/mm^3$. Levels may reach $25,000/mm^3$ during labor.
- Increased fibrin, fibrinogen, and factors VII, VIII, IX, X.

Gastrointestinal System

- Nausea common; vomiting occurs occasionally.
- Ptyalism (excessive salivation) is an occasional problem.
- Intestines and stomach are displaced by uterus.
- Relaxed cardiac sphincter leads to reflux of acidic secretions, resulting in heartburn.
- Delayed gastric emptying leads to constipation.
- Hemorrhoids may develop.

Urinary Tract

- Increased pressure on the bladder from the growing uterus during the first and third trimesters leads to urinary frequency.
- Glomerular filtration rate (GFR) and renal plasma flow (RPF) increase.
- Increased incidence of glycosuria, which may be normal or may indicate gestational diabetes mellitus (see Chapter 2).

Skin and Hair

- Increased pigmentation of areola, nipples, vulva, and linea nigra.
- Facial chloasma, a butterfly-shaped area of pigmentation over the face, may develop. Usually fades after childbirth. Called the "mask of pregnancy."
- Striae or stretch marks may develop on the abdomen, breasts, and thighs.
- Vascular spider nevi, small, bright-red elevations of the skin radiating from central body, may develop.
- Rate of hair growth may decrease.

Musculoskeletal System

- Joints of pelvis relax somewhat.
- Waddling gait develops because of changed center of gravity and accentuated lumbosacral curve.
- Separation of rectus abdominis muscle, called diastasis recti, may occur.

Signs of Pregnancy

Subjective (Presumptive) Changes

- Symptoms experienced by woman.
- May be caused by conditions other than pregnancy.
- Signs include the following: amenorrhea, nausea and vomiting, excessive fatigue, urinary frequency, changes in the breasts, and quickening (mother's perception of fetal movement).

Objective (Probable) Changes

- Signs perceived by the examiner.
- May be caused by conditions other than pregnancy.
- Signs include the following: changes in the pelvic organs such as Goodell's sign, Chadwick's sign, and Hegar's sign (softening of the isthmus, the area between the cervix and the body of the uterus); enlargement of the abdomen; Braxton Hicks contractions; uterine souffle (soft blowing sound heard when auscultating the abdomen, caused by blood pulsating through the placenta); changes in pigmentation of the skin (chloasma, linea nigra); abdominal striae; fetal outline palpable during examination; and positive pregnancy test.

Diagnostic (Positive) Changes

- Signs that are completely objective and caused only by pregnancy.
- Signs include the following: verification of a gestational sac or fetal parts and heartbeat through ultrasonography, as

well as detection of fetal heartbeat and fetal movements by a trained examiner.

Psychologic Responses of the Mother to Pregnancy

Unless the following responses are extreme or exaggerated, they are considered normal. They are related to hormonal changes and to the body's efforts to prepare for childbirth and parenting.

Ambivalence

- Common initially, even if pregnancy is planned.
- Mother may have concerns about her career, her relationship with her partner, financial implications, and role change.
- She may make comments such as, "I thought I wanted a baby, but now I'm not so sure."

Acceptance of Pregnancy

- As acceptance grows, the woman shows a high degree of tolerance for the discomforts she may experience in the first trimester.
- In the second trimester she begins to wear maternity clothes.
- She begins to perceive movement at about 17–20 weeks. She may make comments such as, "Feeling the baby move makes it all seem real" or "It's finally sinking in that I'm going to be a mother."

Introversion

- The expectant woman typically becomes more inwardly focused, less interested in outside activities.
- She is using this time to plan and adjust.
- Her partner may see this as excluding him. She may say, "I never used to like to be alone, but now I like having time to myself just to think and plan."

Mood Swings

- Mood swings from joy to sadness are common and difficult for the woman and her family.

- The woman often feels a great need for love and affection, but her partner, confused by her emotional changes, may react by withdrawing. She may say, "I'm not usually so emotional but lately any little thing can set me off."

Changes in Body Image

- The woman tends to feel somewhat negative about her body as pregnancy progresses.

- Her increasing abdomen coupled with the waddling gait of pregnancy may cause a woman to feel ungainly and unattractive. She may say, "I can't even see my feet anymore" or "I feel as big as a house."

Psychologic Tasks of the Mother

Rubin (1984) identified the following developmental tasks of the mother:

1. *Ensuring safe passage through pregnancy, labor, and birth.* To meet this task she seeks competent prenatal care, practices good health behaviors and self-care activities, reads about childbirth, and gathers information.

2. *Seeking acceptance of this child by others.* The expectant woman seeks to gain support for the coming child from her partner and family. She will also work to help her other children accept the coming baby.

3. *Seeking of commitment and acceptance of self as mother to the infant (binding-in).* After she perceives fetal movement (quickening) the mother begins to form bonds of attachment to the child, and the child becomes more real. The woman may talk about the child as a separate person: "The baby was so active today! I don't think he (or she) appreciated the pizza last night."

4. *Learning to give of one's self on behalf of one's child.* The woman begins to develop patterns of self-denial and

delayed personal gratification to meet the needs of her child. She may, for example, give up smoking or alcohol and make plans to adjust her personal schedule to spend more time with her child.

Critical Terms for Antepartal Assessment

Gravida: Any pregnancy, regardless of duration.

Primigravida: A woman who is pregnant for the first time.

Multigravida: A woman who is pregnant with her second child or any subsequent pregnancy.

Para: Birth after 20 weeks' gestation, regardless of whether the infant is alive or dead.

Multipara: A woman who has had two or more births at more than 20 weeks' gestation.

Note: In clinical practice caregivers often refer to a woman who is pregnant for the first time as a primip (short for primipara). The correct term would actually be nulligravida, but it is seldom used. A woman becomes a primipara after she has had one birth of more than 20 weeks' gestation. Thus the term could be used on postpartum.

Preterm labor: Labor that occurs after 20 weeks but before the completion of 37 weeks of gestation.

Stillbirth: A fetus born dead after 20 weeks' gestation.

Prenatal Client History

Gravida/Para Notation

- Systems are used to describe a woman's pregnancy history.
- Example: Woman pregnant for the first time is gravida 1, para 0 (or G1 P0).
- Example: Woman pregnant for the second time who has one living child born at term and had one miscarriage (also called spontaneous abortion) is gravida 2 para 1 abortion 1 (G2 P1 Ab1).
- Some agencies use a *more detailed* approach using TPAL.

- Gravida means the same as in the previous example; para refers to the number of infants but is further divided to identify the number of term, preterm, abortions, and living children (TPAL).
- Example: Woman pregnant for the first time is gravida 1 para 0000 (sometimes listed as 10000, 1 for gravida, 0000 for para).
- Example: Second woman (described earlier) would be gravida 2 para 1011, for one term infant, no preterm, one abortion, one living child (21011).

Current Pregnancy

- LMP—that is, first day of last normal menstrual period (helps to date pregnancy).
- Presence of any problems or complications such as bleeding.
- Any discomforts, concerns, or questions.

History of Past Pregnancies

- Number of pregnancies, abortions (spontaneous or therapeutic), living children, and complications. (Helps caregivers avoid unintentionally hurtful comments and alerts them to potential problems. For example, a woman with a history of preterm labor is at increased risk for preterm labor.)

Gynecologic History

- Detailed gynecologic history is obtained.
- Include information on contraceptive history (eg, an intrauterine device [IUD] in place is usually removed because it could cause spontaneous abortion).
- Include history of sexually transmitted infections.
- Include history of abnormal Pap smears.

Current and Past Medical History

- Provides information about woman's general state of health and health habits, as well as any medical-surgical conditions that might affect the pregnancy, such as diabetes, heart disease, and sickle cell anemia.

• Note use of alcohol, cigarettes, or drugs; exposure to teratogens; allergies; current medications; blood type and Rh factor; and record of immunizations, especially rubella.

Religious/Cultural/Occupational History

Information is obtained about any religious preferences, cultural influences, and any workplace hazards.

High-Risk Pregnancy

Certain factors in the woman's history place her at increased risk for complications during her current pregnancy. These factors include smoking, maternal age less than 20, previous preterm birth, and so forth. Preexisting medical conditions such as maternal diabetes automatically place the woman in a higher risk category. After the history is obtained, most agencies use a form to rate the number of risk factors and obtain a score. **Women who fall into a high-risk category are monitored more closely for potential complications.**

Partner's History

Information is obtained about the partner's age; health; current and past medical history; use of substances including alcohol, cigarettes, social drugs, and so forth; blood type and Rh factor; occupation; and attitude about the pregnancy.

Initial Prenatal Physical Examination

The nurse is responsible for the following assessments at the initial prenatal examination:

• Vital signs, including temperature, pulse, respirations, and blood pressure (some agencies omit temperature).
• Height and weight.
• Urinalysis (to detect proteinuria, glycosuria, hematuria, and so forth).

- Blood for complete blood count (CBC), including hematocrit (to detect anemia) and differential, Venereal Disease Research Laboratories (VDRL), ABO and Rh typing, Rubella titer (to detect whether the woman is immune to German measles), sickle cell screen for clients of African descent, and other lab tests as ordered.

The nurse then remains in the room to assist the examiner with the physical exam, including the pelvic exam.

Critical Elements of Initial Prenatal Examination

1. **Skin.** Color noted (to detect anemia, cyanosis, jaundice); edema noted (may be normal or could indicate pregnancy-induced hypertension); changes normally associated with pregnancy noted, such as chloasma, linea nigra, and spider nevi.

2. **Neck.** Thyroid assessed, may enlarge slightly during pregnancy; marked enlargement, nodules, and so forth could indicate hyperthyroidism or goiter and are assessed further.

3. **Lungs.** Inspection, palpation, and auscultation should be normal, with no adventitious sounds.

4. **Breasts.** Inspection and palpation performed. Normal changes of pregnancy noted. Orange-peel skin and palpable nodule suggest possible carcinoma; redness indicates mastitis.

5. **Heart.** Rate, rhythm, and heart sounds noted; should be normal. Short systolic murmur common due to increased blood volume.

6. **Abdomen.** Inspection and palpation performed. Liver and spleen not palpable. Shows changes of pregnancy including enlargement and striae.
   a. Fundus (upper portion of uterus) palpable as follows:
      - 10–12 weeks: Slightly above symphysis.
      - 16 weeks: Halfway between symphysis and umbilicus.

- 20 weeks: At umbilicus.
- 28 weeks: Three finger breadths above umbilicus.
- 36 weeks: Just below ensiform cartilage.

b. Fetal heartbeat auscultated as follows:

- 10–12 weeks: Heard with Doppler (rate 120–160 beats/minute).
- 17–20 weeks: Heard with stethoscope.

c. Examiner can palpate fetal movement at 20 weeks' gestation.

7. **Reflexes.** At least brachial and patellar assessed. Hyperreflexia could indicate developing pregnancy-induced hypertension (PIH). (See Procedure: Assessing Deep Tendon Reflexes and Clonus, on page 285. PIH is discussed in Chapter 2.)

8. **Pelvic exam.** External and internal genitals inspected, Pap obtained; gonorrhea culture (and sometimes chlamydia screen) obtained; changes of pregnancy noted, including Chadwick's sign and Goodell's sign. Uterine size evaluated to determine whether size seems appropriate for length of gestation. Ovaries palpated.

9. **Pelvic dimensions.** The following dimensions are considered necessary for vaginal birth (see Figures 1–1, 1–2, and 1–3):

- Pelvic inlet: Diagonal conjugate (extends from lower border of symphysis pubis to sacral promontory) at least 11.5 cm (Figure 1–1).
- Pelvic outlet: Anteroposterior diameter (from lower border of symphysis pubis to tip of sacrum) 9.5–11.5 cm (Figure 1–1).
- Pelvic outlet: Transverse diameter (measured by placing a fist between the ischial tuberosities) 8–10 cm (Figure 1–2).
- Subpubic angle: Obtained by palpating bony structure externally, normally 85–90 degrees (Figure 1–3).
- Mobility of coccyx assessed by pressing on coccyx; it should be mobile.

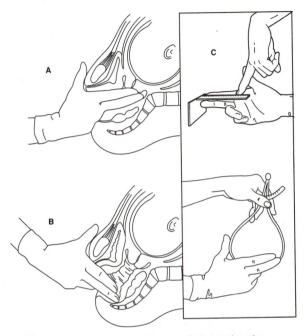

Figure 1–1   Manual measurement of inlet and outlet.
A, Estimation of diagonal conjugate, which extends from the lower border of the symphysis pubis to the sacral promontory. **B,** Estimation of anteroposterior diameter of the outlet, which extends from the lower border of the symphysis pubis to the tip of the sacrum. **C,** Methods that may be used to check manual estimation of anteroposterior measurements.

10. **Rectal exam.** Rashes, lumps, and hemorrhoids noted; woman with hemorrhoids should be assessed for problems with constipation.

Determination of Due Date

The due date (date around which childbirth will occur), also called the estimated date of birth (EDB), estimated date of

Figure 1–2 Use of closed fist to measure outlet. Most examiners know the distance between the first and last proximal knuckles. If not, a measuring device can be used.

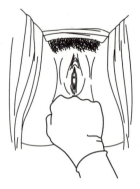

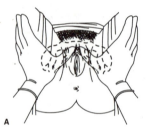

A

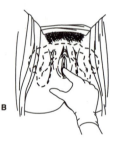

B

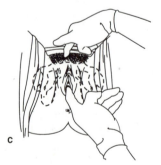

C

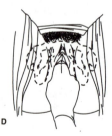

D

Figure 1–3 Evaluation of outlet. **A,** Estimation of suprapubic angle. **B,** Estimation of length of pubic ramus. **C,** Estimation of depth and inclination of pubis. **D,** Estimation of contour of suprapubic angle.

delivery (EDD), or estimated date of confinement (EDC), helps the caregiver determine if the fetus is growing appropriately. It also helps determine whether the start of labor occurs at the correct time or prematurely.

1. **Nägele's rule.** Due date is calculated using a formula called Nägele's rule. To use this formula one begins with the first day of the woman's last menstrual period (LMP), subtracts 3 months, and adds 7 days. For example:

First day of LMP	November 21
Subtract 3 months	−3 months
	August 21
Add 7 days	+7 days
EDB	August 28

   Note: Due date can also be calculated using a *gestational wheel.*

2. **Uterine assessment, or sizing the uterus.** A skilled examiner can determine by bimanual examination if the size of the uterus is appropriate for the weeks of pregnancy. This is an especially valuable technique in the first trimester.

3. **Measurement of fundal height.** After the first trimester the uterus is palpable in the abdomen. Its height can be measured by using a centimeter tape measure to measure the distance from the top of the symphysis pubis to the top of the fundus. Fundal height corresponds well with weeks of gestation, especially between 20 and 31 weeks. For example, 24 cm would suggest 24 weeks' gestation.

4. **Quickening** (perception of fetal movement by the mother). Quickening almost always occurs by 19 to 20 weeks' gestation. Because it may occur any time from 16 to 22 weeks, this is a less specific measure.

5. **Fetal heartbeat.** The heartbeat can be detected with a Doppler by 10–12 weeks' gestation and with a fetoscope by 19–20 weeks' gestation.

6. **Ultrasound.** This procedure can be used to detect a gestational sac in early pregnancy and to determine specific fetal measurements such as biparietal diameter. These measurements are useful in determining gestational age.

Frequency of Prenatal Visits in Normal Pregnancy

- Every 4 weeks for first 28 weeks of gestation.
- Every 2 weeks to week 36.
- After week 36, weekly until birth.

Initial Psychosocial Assessment

The psychosocial assessment helps to determine the woman's attitude about the pregnancy, teaching needs, support systems available to her, cultural or religious preferences, economic status, and living conditions. The following critical nursing assessments require further evaluation and intervention:

- Marked anxiety, apathy, fear, or anger about the pregnancy.
- Isolated home environment without support systems available.
- Language barriers.
- Cultural practices that might endanger the child.
- Long-term family problems.
- Unstable or limited economic status; limited prenatal care.
- Crowded or questionable living conditions.

Care during Regular Prenatal Visits

Critical Nursing Responsibilities

1. **Weigh woman.** During the first trimester a woman gains 3.5–5 lb; during the second and third trimesters she gains about 1 lb per week. Thus, when she is seen every 4 weeks a 4-lb gain is normal. *Be alert for*

   - Inadequate gain: Evaluate reasons, counsel on nutrition.
   - Excessive gain: Often first sign of developing pregnancy-induced hypertension (PIH), a major complication of pregnancy (see Chapter 2 for further assessments).

2. **Monitor vital signs.** Pulse may increase slightly. BP usually decreases slightly toward midpregnancy and gradually returns to normal. Temperature and respirations may be omitted unless adverse symptoms are present. *Be alert for*
   - Rapid pulse: Could indicate anxiety or cardiac problem. Report findings.
   - Elevated BP: A cardinal sign of PIH (see Chapter 2 for further assessments).

3. **Assess for edema.** Some edema of ankles and feet is normal, especially in the last trimester. *Be alert for*
   - Edema of hands, face, and legs—usually related to weight gain and may indicate PIH (see Chapter 2 for further assessments).

4. **Collect dipstick urine specimen.** *Be alert for*
   - Proteinuria 1+. Could indicate PIH (see Chapter 2).
   - Glycosuria: Slight glycosuria may be normal but requires further assessment. Might indicate gestational diabetes mellitus (GDM) (see Chapter 2 for further assessments).

5. **Glucose screen.** Between 24–28 weeks' gestation a 1-hour glucose screen is done. Plasma glucose levels >140 mg/dL indicate the need to complete a 3-hour oral glucose tolerance test (GTT).

6. **Danger signs of pregnancy.** Ask whether the woman is experiencing any of the danger signs of pregnancy (see following discussion).

7. **Discomforts.** Ask about the common discomforts of pregnancy and provide appropriate information (see pages 21–24).

A certified nurse-midwife, nurse practitioner, or physician completes remainder of exam, which includes:

1. Review of history and findings.
2. Assessment of uterine size, measurement of fundal height.
3. Assessment of fetal heartbeat (normal 120–160 bpm) and position.

4. Assessment of deep tendon reflexes (DTRs) and clonus (see Procedure: Assessing Deep Tendon Reflexes and Clonus on page 285).

5. Vaginal exam not repeated until last weeks of pregnancy.

Danger Signs of Pregnancy and Their Possible Causes

Table 1–1 identifies the danger signs of pregnancy and their possible causes. These findings indicate a potentially serious

Table 1–1   Danger Signs in Pregnancy

The woman should report the following danger signs in pregnancy immediately:

Danger Sign	Possible Cause
1. Sudden gush of fluid from vagina	Premature rupture of membranes
2. Vaginal bleeding	Abruptio placentae, placenta previa, lesions of cervix or vagina, "bloody show"
3. Abdominal pain	Premature labor, abruptio placentae
4. Temperature above 38.3°C (101°F) and chills	Infection
5. Dizziness, blurring of vision, double vision, spots before eyes	Hypertension, preeclampsia
6. Persistent vomiting	Hyperemesis gravidarum
7. Severe headache	Hypertension, preeclampsia
8. Edema of hands, face, legs, and feet	Preeclampsia
9. Muscular irritability, convulsions	Preeclampsia, eclampsia
10. Epigastric pain	Preeclampsia-ischemia in major abdominal vessels
11. Oliguria	Renal impairment, decreased fluid intake
12. Dysuria	Urinary tract infection
13. Absence of fetal movement	Maternal medication, obesity, fetal death

problem and require further assessment. The nurse reviews these signs and stresses to the woman the importance of reporting them immediately if they occur. *Discuss them at each prenatal visit.*

Prenatal Nutrition

1. Recommended dietary allowance (RDA) for most nutrients increases.
2. For a woman of normal prepregnant weight, the recommended weight gain is 25–35 lb (11.4–15.9 kg).
3. Pattern of weight gain:
   - First trimester: 3.5–5 lb (1.6–2.3 kg).
   - Second and third trimesters: About 1 lb per week.
   - Caloric increase: Only 300 kcal day. Idea that woman is "eating for two" can lead to excessive weight gain.
4. Overweight women should not diet during pregnancy.
5. In second and third trimesters, further evaluation is indicated for the following:
   - Inadequate gain (less than 2.2 lb [1 kg]/month).
   - Excessive gain (more than 6.6 lb [3 kg]/month).

Critical Information in Counseling about Nutrition

1. Stress the use of the Food Guide Pyramid, including the following:

   Bread, cereal, rice, and pasta: Adults need 6 to 11 servings (1 serving = 1 slice bread, 1 oz dry cereal, 1/2 hamburger roll, 1 tortilla, 1/2 cup pasta, 1/2 cup rice or grits).

   Vegetable group: Adults need 3 to 5 servings (1 serving = 1/2 cup cooked vegetables; 1 cup raw vegetables).

   Fruit group: Adults need 2 to 4 servings (1 serving = 1 medium-sized piece of fruit, 1/2 cup of juice). One serving should be a good source of vitamin C.

Milk, yogurt, cheese group: Adults need 2 to 3 servings (1 serving = 1 cup milk or yogurt, 1.5 oz hard cheese, 2 cups cottage cheese, 1 cup pudding made with milk).

Meat, poultry, fish, dry beans, eggs, and nuts group: Adults need 2 to 3 servings (1 serving = 2 oz cooked lean meat, poultry, or fish; 2 eggs; 1/2 cup cooked legumes [kidney, lima, garbanzo, or soy beans, split peas, and so forth]; 6 oz tofu; 2 oz nuts or seeds; 4 T peanut butter).

Fats, oils, sweets: Use sparingly.

2. To increase diet by 300 kcal, woman should add 2 milk servings and 1 meat or alternate.

3. To get maximum benefit without additional calories, use low-fat dairy products, lean cuts of meat, low-fat cooking methods such as baking or broiling instead of frying, and so forth.

4. Limit extras that have little nutritional value and are high in sugar or fat, such as doughnuts, chips, candy, mayonnaise, and so on.

Nutrition for the Pregnant Adolescent

1. If adolescent is less than 4 years postmenarche, her nutritional needs include the increase for pregnancy (300 kcal) plus the intake necessary for her anticipated weight gain developmentally during the year she is pregnant.

2. Adolescent diets tend to be deficient in iron and calcium. Iron supplements are used and iron-rich foods are encouraged (see following discussion of nutrition for the woman with anemia). Calcium supplements may be necessary, usually 1200 mg daily.

3. Folic acid supplements are given.

4. Many adolescents have a better diet than believed. Thus their eating patterns over several days, not simply one day, should be assessed.

Nutrition for the Pregnant Vegetarian

Lacto-ovovegetarians include milk, dairy products, and eggs in their diet. Some also include fish and poultry. *Lactovegetarians* include dairy products but no eggs. *Vegans* are "pure" vegetarians who do not eat any food from animal sources.

If her diet permits, a woman can obtain adequate complete proteins from dairy products and eggs. Pure vegans must use complementing proteins such as unrefined grains (brown rice, whole wheat), legumes (beans, split peas, lentils), and nuts and seeds (in large quantities). Vegans should take a daily supplement of 4 g of vitamin B_{12}. Vegetarian diets also tend to be low in iron and zinc, and supplementation is often necessary.

Nutrition for the Woman with Anemia

To correct iron deficiency anemia the woman will be given iron supplements. The nurse should explain to her that she can also help herself by the following dietary practices:

- Regularly eat meat, poultry, and fish, which are good sources of iron.
- Consume iron-fortified cereals and breads.
- Iron absorption is increased when vitamin C is taken with meals. Good sources of vitamin C include citrus fruits, strawberries, tomatoes, cantaloupe, broccoli, peppers, and potatoes.
- Select iron-rich vegetables such as spinach, broccoli, dandelion greens, and other green leafy vegetables.
- Use iron pots and pans for cooking.

Relief of the Common Discomforts of Pregnancy

Nausea and Vomiting

- Avoid odors or factors that trigger nausea.
- Eat dry toast or crackers before rising.
- Have small but frequent dry meals with fluids between meals.
- Avoid greasy or highly seasoned foods.
- Drink carbonated beverages or herbal teas (eg, peppermint, chamomile, spearmint).

- May benefit from acupressure wrist bands or acupressure to appropriate pressure points.

Urinary Frequency

- Increase daytime fluid intake; void when the urge is felt.
- Decrease fluid only in the evening to decrease nocturia.

Fatigue

- Plan time for daily nap or rest period.
- Go to bed earlier.
- Seek family assistance with tasks so more time is available to rest.

Breast Tenderness

- Wear well-fitting, supportive bra.

Increased Vaginal Discharge

- Bathe daily but avoid douching, nylon panties, and pantyhose.
- Wear cotton underpants.

Nasal Stuffiness and Epistaxis

- May be unresponsive; cool-air vaporizer may help.
- Avoid nasal sprays and decongestants.

Ptyalism

- Use astringent mouthwash, chew gum, or suck hard candy.

Pyrosis (Heartburn)

- Eat small, frequent meals; avoid overeating or lying down afterward.
- Use low-sodium antacids; avoid sodium bicarbonate.

Ankle Edema

- Dorsiflex foot frequently; elevate legs when sitting or resting.
- Avoid tight garters or constricting bands.

Varicose Veins

- Wear supportive hose and elevate feet frequently.
- Avoid crossing legs at knees, prolonged standing, and garters.

Constipation

- Increase fluid in diet. (Drink at least eight 8-oz glasses daily.)
- Increase fiber. (Increase fruits and vegetables to six servings; choose fresh fruit when possible and include prunes or prune juice; increase grains to six servings and choose unrefined grains, such as whole wheat, brown rice, and bran; include legumes in place of meat.)
- Increase daily exercise to promote peristalsis.

Hemorrhoids

- Avoid constipation and straining to defecate.
- Reinsert into rectum if necessary; treat with topical anesthetics, warm soaks, sitz baths, or ice packs.

Backache

- Use good body mechanics; do pelvic tilt exercise regularly.
- Avoid uncomfortable working heights, high-heeled shoes, lifting heavy loads, and fatigue.

Leg Cramps

- Practice dorsiflexing foot to stretch affected muscle.
- Apply heat to affected muscle.

Faintness

- Avoid prolonged standing in warm area.
- Rise slowly from resting position.

Dyspnea

- Use proper posture when sitting or standing.
- Sleep propped up with pillows if problem occurs at night.

Difficulty Sleeping

- Drink a warm (caffeine-free) beverage before bed.
- Use pillows to provide support for back, between legs, or under upper arm when in a side-lying position.

Flatulence

- Chew food thoroughly and avoid gas-forming food.
- Exercise regularly and maintain normal bowel habits.

Carpal Tunnel Syndrome

- Avoid aggravating hand movements; use splint as prescribed.
- Elevate affected arm.

Monitoring Fetal Activity

- Vigorous fetal activity indicates fetal well-being, whereas a marked decrease in fetal activity may indicate fetal compromise and requires immediate evaluation. Fetal activity may be affected by drugs, cigarette smoking, sound, fetal sleep periods, blood glucose levels, and time of day. It has become accepted practice to teach pregnant women to monitor fetal activity daily beginning at about 27 weeks' gestation.
- The Cardiff Count-to-Ten is a frequently used method to evaluate fetal movement. To complete this self-assessment

the woman begins counting at a specified time daily and counts until 10 fetal movements have occurred. She should contact her caregiver if there are fewer than 10 movements in 3 hours or if it takes much longer each day to note 10 movements. The caregiver will probably order a nonstress test (NST).

Bathing

- Daily bathing, by shower or in a tub, is appropriate. The woman should take care to avoid slipping, especially because of her changed center of gravity. A rubber tub mat helps prevent falls.
- Tub baths are contraindicated in the presence of ruptured membranes or vaginal bleeding to avoid introducing infection.

Employment

Major problems with employment during pregnancy include exposure to fetotoxic hazards, excessive physical strain, overfatigue, medical or pregnancy-related complications, and, in later pregnancy, difficulty with occupations involving balance. Advise the woman who continues working to use breaks and lunch for rest, preferably on her side. Women who stand in place for long periods should dorsiflex their feet and walk around periodically to avoid problems with varicose veins, phlebitis, and edema.

Travel

If no complications exist, there are no restrictions on travel. Travel by plane or train is preferable for long distances. The woman should walk about periodically to avoid phlebitis. If traveling by car she should plan to stop every 2 hours and walk around for 10 minutes. Seat belts should be worn with the lap belt positioned under the abdomen.

Exercise

- Exercise is recommended at least three times per week. Swimming, cycling, walking, and cross-country skiing are good choices.
- Pregnancy is not the time to learn a new or strenuous sport.
- A pregnant woman should wear a supportive bra and appropriate shoes, should avoid hyperthermia, and should take fluids liberally to avoid dehydration.
- The woman should exercise for shorter intervals and should stop when she becomes fatigued.
- To avoid supine hypotensive syndrome she should not lie flat on her back to exercise after the first trimester.
- Dizziness, extreme shortness of breath, tingling and numbness, palpitations, abdominal pain, vaginal bleeding, and abrupt cessation of fetal movement should be reported to her caregiver.

Exercises in Preparation for Childbirth

Teach abdominal tightening; partial, bent-knee sit-ups; Kegel exercises; and tailor sitting.

Sexual Activity

- Change in desire is normal and may vary according to trimester.
- In the first trimester, fatigue, nausea, and breast tenderness may lead to decreased desire in some women. The second trimester may be a time of increased desire, while the third trimester may be a time of decreased desire.
- A woman should avoid lying flat on her back for intercourse after the fourth month to avoid vena caval (aortacaval) syndrome. If that position is preferred she should place a pillow under her right hip to displace the uterus. Change in position, such as side-lying, female superior, or vaginal rear entry, may become necessary as her uterus enlarges.

- In the last weeks of pregnancy orgasms may be more intense and may be followed by uterine cramping.
- **Stress that sexual intercourse is contraindicated once the membranes are ruptured or in the presence of vaginal bleeding to avoid introducing infection.** Women with a history of preterm labor may be advised to avoid intercourse in the third trimester because the oxytocin released with orgasm or with breast stimulation may trigger contractions. Couples who engage in anal intercourse should avoid going from anal penetration to vaginal penetration because of the risk of introducing infection.
- Men may notice a change in their level of desire, too. If a man feels the desire for further sexual release he may need to masturbate, either with his partner or in private.
- The couple can also be encouraged to explore other methods of expressing intimacy and affection, such as stroking, cuddling, and kissing.

Medications, Smoking, and Alcohol

- Women should avoid taking medication—both prescribed and over-the-counter medication—when pregnant. If the need for medication arises, the woman should make certain her caregiver knows she is pregnant.
- Smoking is related to lower birth weight infants and to preterm labor. Women should avoid it as much as possible.
- Alcohol has been linked to neurologic deficits in newborns and to low birth weight. Heavy drinking may lead to fetal alcohol syndrome. Since it is not clear how much alcohol is problematic, it should be avoided. Women should also avoid cocaine, crack, marijuana, and all social and street drugs during pregnancy.

Charting

Most prenatal records are composed of a series of columns for making notations succinctly. These columns include height, weight, blood pressure, urine, fetal heart rate, fundal height, edema, fetal movement, clonus, and so forth. Notations should be made in the comments sections about any deviations from normal, about any teaching done, and about any special procedures. Charting on the prenatal record tends to be especially succinct, as the following example demonstrates:

> Basic four food groups and caloric increases for pregnancy discussed. Handout on prenatal nutrition reviewed and given to client. Reports she is taking prenatal vitamins regularly. States that nausea has decreased and she is walking 2 miles/four times/week. No problems or distress. Will call if symptoms develop. A. Smythe, RN

Assessment of Fetal Well-Being

Ultrasound

- Obstetric ultrasound is done either vaginally or transabdominally, depending on the timing in pregnancy and the purpose of the ultrasound. Ultrasound is generally painless and nonradiating to the woman and fetus; it has no known harmful effects. Serial studies can be done for assessment and comparison.

- Ultrasound can be used for early identification of pregnancy (as early as the 5th or 6th week after LMP); for identification of more than one fetus; to measure biparietal diameter; to detect fetal anomalies, hydramnios (excess amniotic fluid), or oligohydramnios (too little fluid); to locate and grade the placenta; and to observe fetal heart rate, movement, respirations, position and presentation, or fetal death.

Nonstress Test

1. The nonstress test (NST) is used to assess fetal status using an electronic fetal monitor to observe baseline variability and acceleration of fetal heart rate (FHR) with movement. FHR accelerations indicate that the fetal central and autonomic nervous systems have not been affected by decreased oxygen to the fetus.

2. **Procedure.** NST may be done in a clinic or an inpatient setting. The woman is placed in semi-Fowler's position, in a side-lying position, or in a reclining chair. Two belts are placed on the woman's abdomen: one records the FHR, the other records uterine or fetal movement. The fetal monitor begins recording activity. The woman is instructed to press a button on the monitor (or on the uterine belt) each time she feels the fetus move. This causes a mark on the tracing paper. An assessment can then be made as to whether FHR accelerations occurred with each fetal movement.

3. Interpretation of NST results:

   - **Reactive test** shows two or more accelerations of 15 beats/minute, lasting 15 seconds or more, over a period of 20 minutes (Figure 1–4).
   - **Nonreactive test** is one in which the reactive criteria are not met (Figure 1–5).
   - **Unsatisfactory test** is one in which data cannot be interpreted or there is inadequate fetal activity.

4. A reactive NST usually indicates fetal well-being and the test does not need to be repeated for a week. A nonreactive NST indicates the need for further testing.

5. **Nursing interventions.** The nurse explains the procedure, administers the NST, interprets the results, and reports the findings to the physician or certified nurse-midwife. If the fetus is not moving well, it is sometimes helpful to have the mother drink a glass of juice to increase her blood glucose level. This seems to result in increased fetal activity.

   Note: If any decelerations in FHR occur during the procedure, the physician or nurse-midwife should be notified for further evaluation of fetal status.

Biophysical Profile

The biophysical profile (BPP) is a collection of information regarding selected fetal measurements and assessments of the fetus and the amniotic fluid. It includes five variables: fetal breathing movements, body movement, tone, FHR activity,

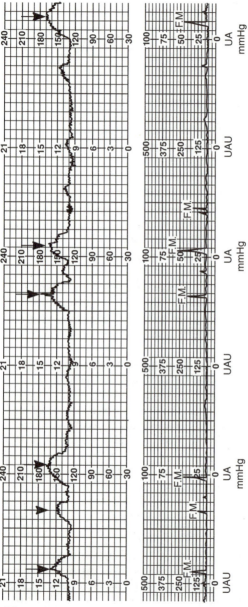

Figure 1–4 Example of a reactive nonstress test (NST). The top portion of the strip is a recording of the FHR. Note that most of the FHR tracing is relatively straight, with some areas that rise from this relatively straight line. These are accelerations. Each small square of the graph paper equals 10 seconds, so each of the indicated accelerations is more than 15 seconds in length. Each of the identified accelerations occurs with a fetal movement (FM), which is recorded on the bottom portion of the strip. The criteria for a reactive NST have been met on this tracing.

30

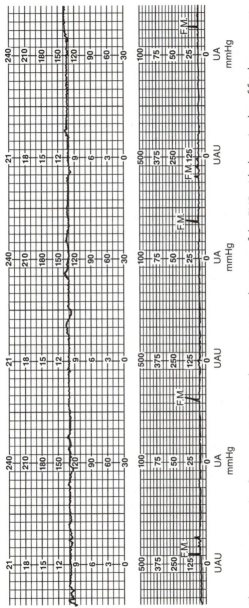

Figure 1–5 Example of a nonreactive NST. There are no accelerations of the FHR with the episodes of fetal movement indicated on the bottom portion of the strip.

and amniotic fluid volume. Table 1–2 identifies scoring techniques and interpretation. Table 1–3 outlines a management protocol.

Amniotic Fluid Analysis (Amniocentesis)

- Amniotic fluid can be withdrawn through a needle inserted through the abdominal wall into the uterus and analyzed to obtain valuable information about fetal status. Amniotic fluid analysis provides genetic information about the fetus and can also be used to determine fetal lung maturity. (See Procedure: Assisting during Amniocentesis, on page 291.)

- Fetal lung maturity can be ascertained by determining the ratio of the phospholipids lecithin and sphingomyelin, the **L/S ratio.** These are two components of surfactant, the substance that lowers the surface tension of the alveoli of the lungs when the newborn exhales, thereby preventing lung collapse. Early in pregnancy the sphingomyelin component is greater than the lecithin, so that the lecithin-to-sphingomyelin (L/S) ratio is low. As pregnancy progresses the lecithin increases. Fetal maturity is indicated by an L/S ratio of 2:1 or greater.

- Delayed lung maturation is often seen in infants born to diabetic mothers. Thus an L/S ratio of 3:1 or higher may be necessary in these infants to ensure lung maturity.

- **Phosphatidylglycerol (PG)**, another phospholipid, appears in the amniotic fluid after about 35 weeks' gestation, and the amount continues to increase to term.

- **Amniotic creatinine** progressively increases with the length of pregnancy, apparently because of increasing fetal muscle mass and maturing fetal renal function. Creatinine levels of 2 mg/dL are associated with fetal maturity.

Table 1–2 Biophysical Profile Scoring: Technique and Interpretation

Biophysical Variable	Normal (Score = 2)	Abnormal (Score = 0)
1. Fetal breathing movements	≥1 episode of ≥30 sec in 30 min	Absent or no episode of ≥30 sec in 30 min
2. Gross body movements	≥3 discrete body/limb movements in 30 min (episodes of active continuous movement considered as single movement)	≤2 episodes of body/limb movements in 30 min
3. Fetal tone	≥1 episode of active extension with return to flexion of fetal limb(s) or trunk; opening and closing of hand considered normal tone	Either slow extension with return to partial extension or movement of limb in full extension or absent fetal movement
4. Reactive fetal heart rate	≥2 episodes of acceleration of ≥15 bpm and of ≥15 sec associated with fetal movement in 20 min	<2 episodes of acceleration of fetal heart rate or acceleration of <15 bpm in 20 min
5. Qualitative amniotic fluid volume	≥1 pocket of fluid measuring ≥1 cm in two perpendicular planes	Either no pockets or a pocket <1 cm in two perpendicular planes

Source: Manning, F. A. et al. (1985). Fetal assessment based on fetal biophysical profile scoring: Experience in 12,620 referred high-risk pregnancies. *American Journal of Obstetrics and Gynecology, 151*(3), 344.

Table 1–3   Management Based on Biophysical Profile Score

Attained Score	Intervention
10 of 10, or 8 of 10, with normal amniotic fluid volume	No intervention needed, normal finding.
8 of 10 with abnormal amniotic fluid volume	If fetal renal function is normal and membranes are intact, delivery is indicated.
6 of 10 with normal amniotic fluid volume	Deliver fetus if it is mature. If immature, repeat test within 24 hours. If score is 6 of 10 or below, deliver fetus.
4 of 10, or 2 of 10, or 1 of 10	Deliver fetus.

Source: Adapted from Manning, F. A. (1990, April 9–12). *The biophysical profile: Contemporary use.* Tenth International Symposium on Perinatal Medicine and Obstetrical Ultrasound, Las Vegas, NV.

References

Rubin, R. (1984). *Maternal identity and the maternal experience.* New York: Springer.

Wheeler, L. (1997). *Nurse-midwifery handbook: A practical guide to prenatal and postpartal care.* Philadelphia: Lippincott.

Chapter 2

The At-Risk Antepartal Client

Diabetes Mellitus

- Condition in which the pancreas does not produce enough insulin to allow necessary carbohydrate metabolism. Glucose does not enter the cells, and they become energy depleted.
- The physiologic changes of pregnancy can drastically alter insulin requirements.
  1. In the first half of pregnancy maternal hormones stimulate increased insulin production by the pancreas and increased tissue response to insulin.
  2. In the second half of pregnancy maternal hormones cause increased resistance to insulin. Concurrently, increased amounts of maternal glucose are being diverted to the fetus.
  3. Any diabetic potential may be influenced by this increased stress on the β-cells of the pancreas.
- Classification
  1. Formerly classified according to pharmacologic treatment as type I (insulin-dependent diabetes mellitus [IDDM]) and type II (non-insulin-dependent diabetes mellitus [NIDDM]).
  2. Newer classification (based on cause) into four main categories: type 1, type 2, other specific types, and gestational diabetes mellitus (GDM).

Gestational Diabetes Mellitus

- GDM refers to diabetes that develops during pregnancy.
- Diabetes screening for GDM in women at average risk:
    1. Done at 24 to 28 weeks' gestation.
    2. 50-g, 1-hour oral glucose tolerance test (GTT) used.
    3. If plasma glucose >130 mg/dL, 3-hour oral GTT indicated.
- Diabetes screening for GDM women at high risk:
    1. Blood glucose screen as soon as possible.
    2. Fasting plasma glucose >126 mg/dL or a casual (any time of the day) plasma glucose >200 mg/dL is diagnostic if confirmed on the following day (American Diabetes Association[ADA], 2000a).
    3. If initial screen is normal, retest at 24–28 weeks.
- Often gestational diabetes can be managed with diet, although some women receive regular insulin as well.

Pregestational Diabetes Mellitus

- Diabetes Mellitus (DM) present before conception.
- Changes in glucose metabolism that result with pregnancy can affect diabetic control and can contribute to possible accelerations of the vascular disease associated with DM.
- Infants of diabetic mothers (IDM) are at greater risk for mortality or morbidity than infants of mothers without diabetes.
- Treatment: insulin only because oral antihyperglycemic agents are teratogenic to the fetus.
- Maternal risks: Hydramnios (excessive volume of amniotic fluid), pregnancy-induced hypertension, ketoacidosis, fetal macrosomia (large-size infant) leading to dystocia (difficult labor), anemia, monilial vaginitis, urinary tract infection (UTI), and retinopathy.
- Fetal-neonatal risks: Intrauterine growth restriction (IUGR), macrosomia, hypoglycemia, respiratory distress syndrome, hyperbilirubinemia, and congenital anomalies.

Management of Diabetes Mellitus in Pregnancy

- Dietary regulation:
  1. Caloric needs of pregnant women are not altered by diabetes—about 30 kcal/kg ideal body weight (IBW) during first trimester and 35 kcal/kg IBW during second and third trimesters (Spellacy, 1999).
  2. Approximately 40% to 50% of calories should come from complex carbohydrates, 15% to 20% from protein, and 30% from fat (Curet, 2000).
  3. These calories are divided among three meals and three snacks.
  4. Bedtime snack is most important because of the risk of hypoglycemia during the night and should contain both protein and complex carbohydrates.
- Glucose monitoring:
  1. Weekly in-office assessment of fasting glucose levels and occasional postprandial checks are generally indicated.
  2. Home monitoring of blood glucose levels four to six times daily.
  3. Optimal range, before meals: 70–100 mg/dL, 2 hours postprandial: <120 mg/dL (ADA, 2000b).
- Insulin administration:
  1. Insulin generally given in multiple injections using human insulin or a fast-acting human analog called Lispro.
  2. Four-dose approach often used with regular insulin or Lispro before each meal and NPH or Lente insulin added at bedtime.
  3. Insulin may also be given by continuous subcutaneous infusion.
  4. *Note:* Oral hypoglycemics are teratogenic and are never used in pregnancy.
- Evaluation of fetal status:
  1. Woman is taught to monitor daily fetal activity (see Chapter 1).

2. Maternal serum alpha-fetoprotein (MSAFP) screening is done at 16 to 20 weeks' gestation.

3. Twice weekly nonstress tests (NSTs) (see Chapter 1) are begun at 32 weeks. Some clinicians delay beginning NSTs until closer to term in women with GDM (Landon, 2000).

4. Biophysical profiles are done in the third trimester to evaluate fetal well-being.

Antepartal Nursing Assessments for Diabetes Mellitus

- Assess urine for glucose and ketones at each prenatal visit.
- Assess results of blood glucose testing for women with diagnosed GDM or pregestational DM.
- Assess for any signs of UTI (dysuria, urgency, frequency, hematuria) or monilial vaginitis (excessive itching, curdy white discharge, dyspareunia).
- Assess woman's understanding of her condition, its treatment, and its implications.
- *Be alert for* hyperglycemia, hypoglycemia, evidence of infection, signs of vascular complications (ulceration of extremities, visual changes, and so forth).

Sample Nursing Diagnoses

- Health-seeking behaviors: Information about GDM related to an expressed desire to learn more about the disease and its implications for the woman and her unborn child.
- Altered family processes related to the client's hospitalization for stabilization of her DM.

Antepartal Nursing Interventions for Diabetes Mellitus

- Obtain serum glucose readings at the specified times (if woman is hospitalized).
- Administer insulin as prescribed. Have a second nurse verify the dosage before administering the insulin.

- Monitor for signs of developing hypoglycemia (caused by too much insulin or too little food): sudden onset (minutes to 1/2 hour), sweating, periodic tingling, disorientation, shakiness, pallor, clammy skin, irritability, hunger, headache, and blurred vision.

  1. If untreated, convulsions and coma may develop.

  2. If they occur, immediately check woman's capillary glucose level (and teach her to do the same following discharge).

  3. Follow agency policy regarding procedure for correcting hypoglycemia for blood glucose >60 mg/dL. The policy may include administering 15 oz milk or 12 oz orange juice or apple juice (Mandeville & Troiano, 1992). If the woman is not alert enough to swallow, give 1 mg glucagon subcutaneously or intramuscularly (IM) and notify physician.

- Monitor for signs of developing hyperglycemia (caused by too much food and too little insulin): typically slow onset, polyuria, polydipsia, dry mouth, increased appetite, fatigue, nausea, hot and flushed skin, rapid and deep breathing, abdominal cramps, acetone breath, headache, drowsiness, depressed reflexes, oliguria or anuria, and stupor or coma.

  1. If hyperglycemia is suspected, obtain frequent measures of blood glucose level; check urine for acetone.

  2. Administer prescribed amount of regular insulin subcutaneously, intravenously, or by a combination of routes.

  3. Replace fluids; measure intake and output (I&O).

- Monitor fetal status including fetal heart rate (FHR) q4h.

- Assist woman with determining fetal movement record daily.

- Do NSTs as ordered while woman is hospitalized.

- Provide appropriate American Diabetes Association (ADA) diet as indicated. Work with dietitian to ensure appropriate teaching is provided for the woman.

- Demonstrate procedure for home monitoring of blood glucose level:
  1. Wash hands thoroughly before finger puncture.
  2. Sides of fingers should be punctured (ends contain more pain-sensitive nerves).
  3. Hanging arm down for 30 seconds before puncture increases blood flow to fingers. Spring-loaded devices are available to make puncture easier.
  4. Cleanse finger with alcohol pad first and allow alcohol to air dry.
  5. Touch blood droplet, not finger, to test pad on strip. Droplet should completely cover the test pad.
  6. If using visual method, wait prescribed time and compare color to color chart. If using a glucose meter, follow directions for use exactly.
  7. Record results and bring record sheet to each prenatal visit.
- Complete client teaching, including the following:
  1. Procedures for home glucose monitoring and insulin administration (if woman is not already familiar with them).
  2. Signs of hypoglycemia and required treatment.
  3. Signs of hyperglycemia and required treatment.
  4. ADA diet.
- Review the following critical aspects of the care you have provided:
  1. Have I administered the correct doses of insulin at the specified times after first determining blood glucose levels?
  2. Have I been alert for any signs of hypoglycemia or hyperglycemia?
  3. Have I monitored FHR and fetal activity carefully and discussed with the woman her perceptions of fetal activity?
  4. Have I assessed the woman's understanding of her DM and answered her questions? Have I given her opportunities to practice specific skills as necessary?

5. Have I ensured that the woman is eating the appropriate meals?

Evaluation

- The woman is able to discuss her condition and its possible impact on her pregnancy.
- The woman participates in developing a health care regimen to meet her needs and follows it throughout pregnancy.
- The woman avoids developing hypoglycemia or hyperglycemia; if it does develop, therapy is successful in correcting it without complications.
- The woman gives birth to a healthy newborn.

Preeclampsia-Eclampsia during the Antepartal Period

- Preeclampsia-eclampsia (also called pregnancy-induced hypertension [PIH]) is the most common hypertensive disorder in pregnancy.
- It is characterized by the development of hypertension, proteinuria, and edema.
- The definition of preeclampsia is
  1. A blood pressure (BP) of 140/90 mm Hg during the second half of pregnancy in a previously normotensive woman.
  2. An increase in systolic BP of 30 mm Hg and/or of diastolic BP of 15 mm Hg over baseline also defines PIH.
  3. These blood pressure changes must be noted on at least two occasions 6 hours or more apart for the diagnosis to be made.
- **Mild preeclampsia** is characterized by
  1. BP of 140/90 or +30/+15 over baseline on two occasions at least 6 hours apart.
  2. Generalized edema of the face, hands, legs, and ankles, which is usually associated with a weight gain of more than 1 lb/week.

    3. Proteinuria of 1+ to 2+ on dipstick (less than 5 g in 24 hours).

- **Severe preeclampsia** is characterized by
    1. BP of 160/110 on two occasions at least 6 hours apart while the woman is on bed rest.
    2. Proteinuria >5 g in 24 hours (3+ to 4+ dipstick).
    3. Oliguria (urine output <400 mL/24 hours).
    4. Headache.
    5. Blurred vision, scotomata (spots before the eyes), and retinal edema on funduscopy (retinas appear wet and glistening).
    6. Pulmonary edema.
    7. Hyperreflexia.
    8. Irritability.
    9. Epigastric pain.

- **Eclampsia** is characterized by
    1. Grand mal seizure, which may be preceded by an elevated temperature as high as 38.4°C (101°F), or the temperature may remain normal.
    2. The woman may have just one seizure or from 2 to 20 or more.
    3. Symptoms may increase in severity: BP of 180/110 or higher, 4+ proteinuria, oliguria or anuria, and increased neurologic symptoms such as decreased sensorium or coma.

- Maternal risks with preeclampsia-eclampsia:
    1. Retinal detachment.
    2. Central nervous system changes including hyperreflexia and seizure.
    3. HELLP syndrome (**h**emolysis, **e**levated **l**iver enzymes, and **l**ow **p**latelet count). (*Note:* Women who experience HELLP, a multiple organ failure syndrome, and their offspring have high morbidity and mortality rates.)

- Fetal-neonatal risks:
    1. Prematurity.

2. Intrauterine growth restriction (IUGR).

3. Oversedation at birth because of maternal medications.

4. Mortality rates of 10% with preeclampsia and 20% with eclampsia.

Antepartal Management of Preeclampsia-Eclampsia

Mild Preeclampsia

- May be managed at home.
- Promotion of good placental and renal perfusion:
  1. Frequent rest periods during the day in a side-lying position.
  2. Specific guidelines regarding rest periods may be given, including the amount of time in each rest period, number of rest periods daily, and the activities during the day that are advisable or should be avoided.
  3. The more specific the guidelines, the more likely that the woman will clearly understand the information and restrictions.
- Dietary modifications:
  1. Diet should be high in protein (80–100 g/day, or 1.5 g/kg/day).
  2. Sodium intake should be moderate, not exceeding 6 g/day.
- Evaluation of fetal status:
  1. NSTs and/or fetal biophysical profile done weekly.
  2. Additional tests include serial ultrasounds to evaluate fetal growth, amniocentesis to determine fetal lung maturity, and a contraction stress test if nonstress test results indicate a need.
- Evaluation of maternal well-being:
  1. Woman is seen every 1 to 2 weeks.
  2. Taught to identify signs of a worsening condition.
  3. Does home blood pressure monitoring daily.

Severe Preeclampsia

- Hospitalization necessary.
- Promotion of maternal well-being:
  1. Complete bed rest in left lateral position, which decreases pressure on vena cava, thereby increasing venous perfusion. Improved renal blood flow helps decrease angiotensin II levels, promotes diuresis, and lowers blood pressure.
  2. High protein, moderate sodium diet is continued.
  3. The woman is weighed daily (to detect edema) and evaluated for evidence of a change in condition through assessment of BP, TPR, deep tendon reflexes (DTRs) and clonus, edema (generalized and pitting), presence of headache, visual disturbances, and epigastric pain.
- Evaluation of laboratory data:
  1. Daily hematocrit (rising value may be associated with decreasing vascular volume).
  2. Daily liver enzyme testing including SGOT, SGPT, and LDH (a rise in these tests correlates with a worsening condition).
  3. Daily uric acid and BUN (reflect renal status).
  4. Platelet counts every 2 to 3 days if over 100,000/mm^3; daily if under 100,000/mm^3.

     (*Note:* Platelet count may be included in preeclamptic or disseminated intravascular coagulation [DIC] screen, which also determines prothrombin time, partial thromboplastin time, and fibrinogen and fibrin split products.) Platelet transfusions are indicated if the platelet count is below 20,000/mm^3.
- Medication therapy:
  1. Magnesium sulfate is the treatment of choice for preventing convulsion (see Drug Guide: Magnesium Sulfate, on page 273).
  2. Sedation with phenobarbital 30–60 mg po q6h may be indicated. (Some physicians prefer diazepam [Valium].)

3. An antihypertensive such as hydralazine (Apresoline) or labetalol (Normodyne) may be used if the diastolic pressure is 110 mm Hg or above.

- Fluid and electrolytes are replaced as necessary based on the status of the woman.

Eclampsia

- Actions taken to control seizure may include bolus of magnesium sulfate, sedatives if necessary, and dilantin for seizure prevention.
- The therapies discussed previously are continued.
- The airway is maintained.
- Woman is monitored for pulmonary edema, which may be treated with furosemide (Lasix).
- Digitalis may be given for circulatory failure.
- The woman may be transferred to an intensive care unit.

Antepartal Nursing Assessments for Preeclampsia-Eclampsia

- Assess BP, pulse, and respirations q1–4h and more frequently if indicated.
- Assess temperature q4h unless elevated, then q2h.
- Assess FHR when maternal vital signs (VS) are assessed or continuously with an electronic fetal monitor.
- Assess intake and urinary output hourly or q4h. Output should be 700 mL/24 hr or greater, or at least 30 mL/hr.
- Assess urinary protein by dipstick of each urine specimen or a specimen from an indwelling bladder catheter.
  Assessment technique: A small sample of urine is collected in a urine specimen bottle or in a syringe. A few drops of urine are placed on the treated section of the dipstick. The color of the treated urine is compared to samples on the dipstick container after a specified period of time. See dipstick container for specific instructions.
- Assess urine specific gravity.
- Assess for evidence of edema.

Assessment technique: Assess for pitting edema by pressing over bony areas, usually over the shin. After pressing with one fingertip for 3 to 5 seconds, evaluate the resulting depression. A slight depression is 1+; a pit 1 inch deep is 4+.

- Assess daily weight.

  Assessment technique: Use the same scales each day; weigh at the same time each day with the woman in similar clothing.

- Assess DTRs. Assess for clonus. (See Procedure: Assessing Deep Tendon Reflexes and Clonus, on page 285.)

- Assess breath sounds; rales will be heard if pulmonary edema is developing.

- Assess laboratory results.

- Assess woman's coping responses, level of understanding regarding her condition, and emotional status.

- See Drug Guide: Magnesium Sulfate, on page 273, for specific nursing assessments during $MgSO_4$ therapy.

- *Be alert for* signs of worsening condition (increasing BP, headache, scotomata, increasing edema [especially of hands and face], disorientation, epigastric pain, pitting edema) and signs of $MgSO_4$ toxicity (respirations <12–14/minute, diminished or absent reflexes, urine output <100 mL in 4-hour period).

Sample Nursing Diagnoses

- Fluid volume deficit related to fluid shift from intravascular to extravascular space secondary to vasospasm.

- Risk for injury related to possibility of convulsion secondary to cerebral vasospasm or edema.

- Health-seeking behaviors: Information about preeclampsia related to an expressed desire to understand her condition and its implications.

Antepartal Nursing Interventions for Preeclampsia-Eclampsia

If the woman is managed at home:

- Teach the woman and her support person how to assess BP. Include positioning and specifics of the procedure.

Assist them in developing a chart to record the findings. Instruct them about findings that should be reported to the physician.

- Provide teaching about the rest period regimen. Explain the purpose of the side-lying position.

If the woman is hospitalized:

- Monitor maternal BP, pulse and respirations, DTRs and clonus, and FHR q2–4h.
- Monitor oral temperature q4h unless elevated, then q2h.
- Weigh daily.
- Monitor intake and output. Output should be at least 30 mL/hr. Specific gravity of readings >1.040 indicate oliguria.
- Monitor urine for proteinuria and specific gravity with each voiding or hourly if an indwelling catheter is in place.
- Monitor for signs of worsening condition including headache, visual disturbances, epigastric pain, and change in level of consciousness at least q4h.
- Encourage woman to maintain a side-lying position.
- Provide emotional support and teaching regarding condition and treatment plan.
- Administer $MgSO_4$ and other medications as ordered. Monitor for evidence of effectiveness or toxicity.
- Provide a quiet, restful environment with limited visitors.
- Pad side rails and take seizure precautions.
- Review the following aspects of the care you have provided:
  1. What is the woman's response to the medications? Am I seeing any potential side effects?
  2. Is there a change in her ability to talk? Does she seem more irritable? Confused?
  3. Is she complaining of headache or other symptoms that indicate a worsening condition?
  4. Is the baby moving as much? Is FHR in normal range (120–160 beats/minute)?
  5. Positioning on which side produces the best results in fetal heart rate? Urine output? What can I do to help

the woman maintain that position? A back rub?
Pillows?

6. Have I taken necessary safety precautions, including
   padded side rails, quiet environment, and calcium gluconate (magnesium sulfate antagonist) available?

Sample Nurse's Charting

1600: BP stable at 142/96, P 88, R 18, T 98.4F. FHR 138.
Lungs clear to auscultation. DTRs, patellar and brachial, 2+
with no clonus. Pitting edema 1+ in legs, some swelling of
fingers—rings snug. Slight periorbital edema evident. Urine
S.G. 1.034; hourly output 40 mL/hr through indwelling bladder catheter. 2+ proteinuria. $MgSO_4$ maintenance dose running at 2 g/hr per infusion pump. No edema, redness, or c/o discomfort at infusion site. Continuous EFM with FHR baseline
140–146, LTV average, STV present. Accelerations of 20 bpm
for 20 sec noted with fetal movement. No decelerations noted.
Client drowsy, responsive, oriented. States she has a slight
headache but denies epigastric pain or visual changes. Resting
quietly on her L side. Side rails padded and up. A. Smythe, RN

Evaluation

- The woman is able to explain preeclampsia-eclampsia, its
  implications for her pregnancy, the treatment regimen,
  and possible complications.
- The woman does not have any eclamptic convulsions.
- The woman and her caregivers detect any evidence of
  increasing severity of the disease or possible complications
  early so that appropriate treatment measures can be
  instituted.
- The woman gives birth to a healthy newborn.

Preterm Labor

- Labor that occurs between 20 and 37 completed weeks of
  gestation is referred to as *preterm labor*.
- It may result from maternal factors such as cardiovascular
  or renal disease, PIH, diabetes, abdominal surgery during

pregnancy, a blow to the abdomen, uterine anomalies, cervical incompetence, DES exposure, history of cone biopsy, and maternal infection.

- Fetal factors include multiple pregnancy, hydramnios, and fetal infection, and placental factors include placenta previa and abruptio placentae.

- The major maternal risks involve psychologic stress related to the woman's concern for her unborn child and physiologic side effects of the drugs used to stop labor.

- Fetal-neonatal risks are those related to the effects of prematurity.

Management of Preterm Labor

- Confirmation of diagnosis:
    1. A diagnosis of preterm labor is made if the gestation is between 20 and 37 completed weeks, if there are documented uterine contractions (four in 20 minutes or eight in 60 minutes), and ruptured membranes.
    2. If the membranes are not ruptured one of the following must be present: 80% cervical effacement, documented cervical changes, or 2 cm dilatation.

- Tests to screen high-risk women for preterm labor:
    1. **Fetal fibronectin (fFN).** Fetal fibronectin is a protein normally found in fetal membranes and decidua early in pregnancy, but not between 18 and 36 weeks' gestation. Positive fFN test (fFN in cervicovaginal fluid) between 18 and 36 weeks indicates increased risk; negative test predicts no preterm birth within 7 days (Chez, 1999).
    2. **Salivary estriol.** Maternal estriol levels rise about 3 weeks before birth, whether preterm or term. Salivary estriols help predict preterm birth after about 30 weeks' gestation.
    3. **Transvaginal ultrasound (TVS)**. Length of the cervix can be measured using an ultrasound probe inserted into the vagina. A cervix shorter than 25 mm prior to term is generally abnormal.

- Any medical conditions that may contribute to preterm labor should be treated.
- Mild symptoms may be treated with bed rest and hydration per infusion.
- If labor continues or if symptoms are severe, tocolysis (use of medication to stop labor) is begun.
- Tocolytics currently used to arrest preterm labor include magnesium sulfate, β-adrenergic agonists (also called β-mimetics), prostaglandin synthetase inhibitors (eg, indomethacin [Indocin]), and calcium channel blockers (eg, nifedipine).
  1. Magnesium sulfate is effective and has fewer side effects than the β-adrenergics. A loading dose of 4–6 g is administered IV over 20 minutes. A maintenance dose of 1–4 g/hour via infusion pump is then used until contractions cease (Creasy & Iams, 1999).
  2. Maternal serum level of 6–8 mg/dL is the effective range for tocolysis (see Drug Guide: Magnesium Sulfate, on page 273).
  3. The β-mimetics used include ritodrine (Yutopar), which has been approved by the U.S. Food and Drug Administration (FDA), and terbutaline (Brethine), which is not FDA approved for use in preterm labor but has become increasingly popular because it is effective and less expensive than ritodrine. Terbutaline is administered intravenously until uterine activity ceases.
- Betamethasone, an antenatal corticosteroid, may be given to the mother to help promote fetal lung maturation.

Nursing Assessments for Preterm Labor

- Assess carefully for evidence of complications or side effects from tocolysis including tachycardia, palpitations, nervousness, nausea and vomiting, headache, and hypotension.
- *Be alert for* evidence of pulmonary edema, the most serious complication. Signs include shortness of breath, chest tightness, dyspnea, rales, and rhonchi.

- Assess for symptoms of magnesium toxicity in women receiving magnesium sulfate, including respirations <12/minute, diminished or absent DTRs, and urine output <100 mL in 4-hour period.

Sample Nursing Diagnoses

- Knowledge deficit related to lack of information about causes, identification, and treatment of preterm labor.
- Fear related to the risks of early labor and birth.

Nursing Interventions for Preterm Labor

Home Care

- Instruct women at risk about the signs and symptoms of preterm labor, which include the following:
  1. Uterine contractions occurring q10min or more frequently.
  2. Mild menstrual-like cramps felt low in the abdomen or abdominal cramping with or without diarrhea.
  3. Feelings of pelvic pressure that may feel like the baby pressing down. The pressure may be constant or intermittent.
  4. Constant or intermittent low backache.
  5. A sudden change in vaginal discharge (an increase in amount, or a change to more clear and watery, or a pinkish tinge).
  6. Instruct women on a home monitoring program that they will use a home uterine activity monitor to record and transmit uterine contractile activity via the phone once or twice daily to a nurse specially trained in assessing the signs and symptoms of preterm labor. The nurse uses the data received and the woman's reports of symptoms to evaluate the risk of preterm labor on a daily basis.
- Teach the at-risk woman who is not on a preterm home monitoring program to evaluate contraction activity once or twice daily.
  1. Instruct her to lie on her side and place her fingertips on the fundus of the uterus.

2. She checks for contractions (hardening of the fundus) for about 1 hour.

3. Occasional contractions are probably normal Braxton Hicks contractions.

- If the woman experiences contractions every 10 minutes or any of the previously identified signs of labor, instruct her to do the following:

    1. Empty her bladder and lie down, preferably on her left side.

    2. Drink three to four 8-oz cups of fluid.

    3. Palpate for uterine contractions.

    4. Rest for 30 minutes after symptoms have subsided and gradually resume activity.

    5. Call her health care provider if symptoms persist, even if uterine contractions are not palpable.

Hospital Care

- Encourage bed rest in a side-lying position as much as possible.

- Monitor BP, pulse, and respirations as ordered, especially when on tocolytic therapy.

- Maintain continuous electronic monitoring of FHR and uterine contractions if ordered (see Chapter 3) and evaluate results.

- Monitor intake and output.

- Administer betamethasone as ordered (see Drug Guide, page 268).

- Explain procedures to the woman and her partner; answer questions and provide emotional support.

- Review the following critical aspects of the care you have provided:

    1. What is the woman's response to the tocolysis? Is she showing any side effects of the medication?

    2. Is she still having contractions? Have they increased or lessened? Is she showing other signs of labor?

    3. What is the fetus's response?

4. What position is most effective? Are there nursing measures I can use to help her tolerate the side-lying position and the effects of tocolysis?

5. How is she coping emotionally? Have I spent enough time helping her to cope with the stress of the situation?

Evaluation

- The woman is able to discuss the cause, identification, and treatment of preterm labor.

- The woman can describe self-care measures and can identify characteristics that should be reported to her caregiver.

- The woman and her baby have a safe labor and birth.

Placenta Previa in the Antepartal Period

- In placenta previa the placenta is implanted in the lower uterine segment instead of the upper portion of the uterus. As the lower uterine segment contracts and dilates in the later weeks of pregnancy, the villi are torn from the uterine wall and bleeding results.

- If the placenta previa is complete, the placenta totally covers the internal cervical os.

- In partial placenta previa, a portion of the os is covered.

- Maternal risks are related to the possibility of hemorrhage and to psychologic stress resulting from concern about fetal well-being.

- Fetal-neonatal risks are related to the extent of the placenta previa. If a severe bleeding episode occurs the fetus often suffers fetal distress. Fetal demise is also a possibility if the condition is not diagnosed in a timely manner.

Antepartal Management of Placenta Previa

- **Diagnosis.** Diagnosis is made based on a history of painless, bright-red vaginal bleeding, especially in the third trimester. The initial bleeding episode may be light but is often followed by more severe bleeding. Diagnosis is confirmed with ultrasound to localize the placenta.

• **Expectant management.** If <37 weeks' gestation, expectant management is used to delay birth to allow the fetus to mature. This includes

1. Bed rest.
2. No rectal or vaginal exams.
3. Monitoring of bleeding.
4. Ongoing assessment of fetal status with external monitor.
5. Monitoring of vital signs.
6. Laboratory evaluation (hemoglobin, hematocrit, Rh factor, urinalysis).
7. Two units of cross-matched blood are kept available for transfusion.

• If the previa is partial or if the placenta is simply low lying, vaginal birth may be attempted.
• **Emergency management.** If severe bleeding occurs or evidence of fetal distress develops, a cesarean is performed.

Antepartal Nursing Assessments for Placenta Previa

• Assess woman regularly for evidence of vaginal bleeding. If bleeding is present, note the amount and character.
• Assess for signs of shock if bleeding is present (decreased blood pressure, increased pulse, cool clammy skin, pallor, decreased hematocrit, urine output <30 mL/hour).
• Assess for uterine contractility and signs of labor. *Word of caution:* Vaginal exams may trigger a major bleeding episode and are contraindicated.
• Assess woman's understanding of her condition, its implications, and treatment options.
• Assess fetal status. During bleeding episode, continuous electronic fetal monitoring is used; when no bleeding is present, an electronic fetal monitoring strip is run, usually q4h (timing may vary according to agency policy).

Sample Nursing Diagnoses

- Altered tissue perfusion (placental) related to blood loss.
- Fear related to concern for own personal well-being and that of baby.

Antepartal Nursing Interventions for Placenta Previa

- Carry out ongoing monitoring of maternal and fetal status including VS, evidence of bleeding, urinary output, electronic monitor tracing, and signs of labor.
- Explain procedures to woman and her family.
- Administer IV fluids or blood products as ordered.
- Review the following critical aspects of care you have provided:
  1. Have I questioned the woman about bleeding? If bleeding is present, have I assessed quantity carefully?
  2. Have I carefully monitored fetal status? Any signs of tachycardia? Decelerations?
  3. Have I been alert for any changes in the woman's status? Any signs of labor? Any changes she has noted?
  4. Have I implemented measures to help the woman be comfortable on bed rest—back rubs, positioning with pillows, diversionary activities?

Evaluation

- The woman's condition remains stable or bleeding is detected promptly and therapy is begun.
- The woman and her baby have a safe labor and birth.

Additional Complications

Table 2–1 describes additional complications the nurse may encounter.

Table 2–1 Selected Complications during Pregnancy

Acquired Immunodeficiency Syndrome (AIDS)

Condition/Overview	Signs/Symptoms/Risk	Medical Therapy	Nursing Interventions
AIDS, caused by the human immunodeficiency virus (HIV), is a multisystem disorder that enters the body through blood, blood products, and body fluids such as semen, vaginal fluid, and urine. HIV affects T cells, thereby depressing the body's immune response. The highest incidence of AIDS occurs in homosexual or bisexual men, heterosexual partners of persons with AIDS, IV drug users, hemophiliacs, and fetuses of women at risk or HIV positive. Persons generally test positive for HIV within 6 to 12 weeks of exposure but may remain asymptomatic for 5 to 11 years or more. In the U.S. the	The following women are considered at risk for AIDS: prostitutes; women with a history of sexually transmitted infection; IV drug users; partners (currently or previously) of IV drug users, bisexual men, hemophiliacs, or those who test positive for HIV. Women with AIDS may have any of the following: malaise, weight loss, lymphadenopathy, diarrhea, fever, neurologic dysfunction, immunodeficiency, esophageal candidiasis, herpes simplex virus, vaginal *Candida* infections, and cervical disease. Maternal risks: Complications such as intrapartal or postpartal	Currently there is no definitive therapy for AIDS, although a variety of drugs are available that delay the onset of symptoms. Zidovudine (ZDV) is primary treatment for pregnant women. Current goal is to detect women at risk and educate the public about the spread of AIDS. Women at risk who are pregnant or planning a pregnancy should be offered HIV antibody testing. Women who test positive should be counseled about the implications for themselves and the fetus/newborn. They may be offered a therapeutic abortion. Women who continue pregnancy need excellent	1. Assess history for risk factors. 2. Provide clear information about AIDS, ZDV therapy, and the implications for the woman, her partner, and a child should the woman become pregnant. 3. Monitor asymptomatic pregnant woman for nonspecific symptoms such as fever, weight loss, persistent candidiasis (vaginal yeast infection or thrush in mouth), diarrhea, cough, skin lesions. 4. Implement appropriate isolation procedures including use of disposable

vast majority of pediatric AIDS cases have resulted from perinatal transmission from mother to child.

hemorrhage, postpartal infection, poor wound healing, and infections of the GI tract. Fetal-neonatal risks: Risk of transmission from HIV-positive mother to fetus is about 25%. When pregnant women receive ZDV risk decreases to 5%. Infected infant often asymptomatic at birth; onset of symptoms usually occurs between 9 and 18 months. Facial characteristics that may indicate the newborn has been infected early in utero with HIV include microcephaly; patulous lips; prominent, boxlike forehead; increased distance between inner canthus of eyes; flattened nasal bridge.

prenatal care with attention to psychosocial and teaching needs.

latex gloves when in contact with nonintact skin, mucous membranes, or body fluids (changing chux, diapers, peripads; starting IV, drawing blood); use of protective covering such as plastic apron and glasses or eye shield when contamination from splashing may occur (vaginal exam, vaginal or caesarean birth, suctioning, care of newborn before initial bath). (Consult unit procedure manual for further specifics.)

5. Provide emotional support and nonjudgmental attitude; preserve confidentiality.

(Continued)

Table 2–1 Selected Complications during Pregnancy (continued)

Condition/Overview	Signs/Symptoms/Risk	Medical Therapy	Nursing Interventions
Chlamydia Sexually transmitted infection caused by *Chlamydia trachomatis*, often found in association with gonorrhea.	Women are often asymptomatic. Symptoms may include thin or purulent vaginal discharge, frequency and burning with urination, or lower abdominal pain. Infant of woman with untreated chlamydia is at risk for newborn conjunctivitis, chlamydial pneumonia, preterm birth, or fetal demise.	Nonpregnant women treated with tetracycline. Because this medication may permanently discolor fetal teeth, pregnant women are treated with erythromycin ethyl succinate. Erythromycin eye ointment (but not silver nitrate) can prevent conjunctivitis in the newborn.	1. Review signs and symptoms; explain importance of taking entire dose of medication.
Gonorrhea Sexually transmitted infection caused by *Neisseria gonorrhoeae*.	Majority of women are asymptomatic; disease often diagnosed during routine prenatal cervical culture. If symptoms are present, they may include purulent vaginal	Pregnant women are treated with ceftriaxone plus erythromycin (Centers for Disease Control and Prevention [CDC], 1998). If the woman is allergic to ceftriaxone,	1. Review medication purpose, side effects. 2. Explain that untreated gonorrhea may result in pelvic inflammatory disease and infertility.

	discharge, dysuria, urinary frequency, inflammation and swelling of vulva. Cervix may appear eroded. Infection at time of birth may cause ophthalmia neonatorum in the newborn.	spectinomycin is used. All sexual partners are treated.	3. Discuss safe sexual practices.
Syphilis Sexually transmitted infection caused by the spirochete *Treponema pallidum.*	Primary stage: Chancre, slight fever, malaise. Chancre lasts about 4 weeks, then disappears. Secondary stage: Occurs 6 weeks to 6 months after infection. Skin eruptions (condyloma lata); also symptoms of acute arthritis, liver enlargement, iritis, chronic sore throat with hoarseness.	For syphilis less than 1 year in duration: 2.4 million U benzathine penicillin G IM. For syphilis of more than 1 year's duration: 2.4 million U benzathine penicillin G once a week for 3 weeks. Sexual partners should also be screened and treated.	1. Explain the risk factors and long-term effects if syphilis is not treated. 2. Explain implications for fetus/neonate. 3. Stress importance of receiving all three doses if syphilis is greater than 1 year in duration. *(Continued)*

Table 2–1 Selected Complications during Pregnancy *(continued)*

Condition/Overview	Signs/Symptoms/Risk	Medical Therapy	Nursing Interventions
	Diagnosed by blood tests such as VDRL, RPR, FTA-ABS. Dark-field exam for spirochetes may be done. May be passed transplacentally to fetus. If untreated, one of the following can occur: second-trimester abortion, stillborn infant at term, congenitally infected infant, uninfected live infant.		
TORCH The TORCH group of infectious diseases may cause serious harm to fetus. They include toxoplasmosis (TO), rubella (R), cytomegalic inclusion disease (C), and herpes genitalis (H).	**Toxoplasmosis** results in a mild infection in adults but is associated with an increased risk of spontaneous abortion, prematurity, stillbirth, neonatal death, and disorders including microcephaly, hydrocephalus, convulsions, blindness,	**Toxoplasmosis:** Goal is to identify women at risk. Diagnosis made using serologic testing, physical findings and history. Treatment includes sulfadiazine, pyrimethamine, and spiramycin. If toxoplasmosis is diagnosed	**Toxoplasmosis:** Explain methods of prevention to childbearing woman. She should avoid poorly cooked or raw meat, especially pork, beef, and lamb. Fruits and vegetables should be washed. Litter box should be cleaned frequently

Some sources identify the "O" as "other infections." Exposure of the woman during the first 12 weeks of pregnancy may cause developmental anomalies.

Toxoplasmosis is caused by a protozoan and transmitted by eating raw or poorly cooked meat or by exposure to feces of infected cats. Innocuous in adults.

Rubella or German measles is caused by a virus.

Cytomegalic inclusion disease (CID), caused by the cytomegalovirus (CMV), is the most prevalent infection of the TORCH group. Chronic persistent infection with viral

deafness, and mental retardation.

Rubella exposure in the first trimester is associated with spontaneous abortion, congenital heart disease, intrauterine growth restriction, cataracts, mental retardation, and cerebral palsy. Infection in the second trimester is most often associated with permanent hearing impairment in the newborn.

CID may cause fetal death; in neonates it is associated with microcephaly, cerebral palsy, mental retardation, and so forth. Subclinical infections may cause neurologic and

before 20 weeks' gestation, therapeutic abortion may be offered because damage to the fetus tends to be more severe than if the disease is diagnosed later in pregnancy.

Rubella: Best therapy is prevention by vaccination. Women of childbearing age should be tested for immunity and vaccinated if susceptible. HAI titer of 1:16 or greater indicates immunity. Pregnant women are not vaccinated but will be offered vaccination postpartum. If infection occurs in first trimester, woman will be offered a therapeutic abortion.

by someone else, and woman should wear gloves when gardening.
Rubella: Assess for signs of rubella infection (maculopapular rash, lymphadenopathy, muscular achiness, joint pain). Provide emotional support and objective information for couples contemplating therapeutic abortion.
CID: Provide emotional support and objective information.
Herpes genitalis: Provide information about the disease and its spread. Advise woman to inform future health care providers of her infection. A

(Continued)

61

Table 2–1 Selected Complications during Pregnancy *(continued)*

Condition/Overview	Signs/Symptoms/Risk	Medical Therapy	Nursing Interventions
shedding for years. Usually is asymptomatic in adults and children. **Herpes genitalis,** caused by herpes simplex virus type 2 (HSV-2), is a chronic recurring infection that causes painful lesions in the genital area and is transmitted by sexual contact.	hearing problems that may go unrecognized for months or years. **Herpes genitalis** may cause spontaneous abortion if active HSV-2 infection occurs in first trimester. Highest risk of infection for newborn who is born vaginally when mother has active HSV-2 in her vagina. Risk of neonatal death, permanent brain damage, characteristic skin lesions.	**CID:** Diagnosis is confirmed by serologic tests to detect CMV antibodies. No effective treatment is available at this time. **Herpes genitalis:** The American College of Obstetricians and Gynecologists (ACOG, 1999) recommends antiviral therapy for women with primary HSV infection during pregnancy to decrease viral shedding and promote healing. Three medications are available: acyclovir, valaclovir, and famciclovir. Women with recurrent infection may also be treated with antiviral therapy. Vaginal birth is preferred if there is no evidence of genital	possible association exists between herpes and cervical cancer. Thus women should understand importance of yearly Pap smears. Provide emotional support and nonjudgmental attitude.

infection. If there are any lesions or prodromal symptoms such as vulvar pain or burning, caesarean birth is indicated. Women with active HSV infection and ruptured membranes should give birth by caesarean as soon as possible.

Following diagnosis, management involves a team approach to provide care for woman and fetus/neonate. Hospitalization may be necessary to achieve detoxification. "Cold turkey" withdrawal is not advised because of risk to fetus. Urine screening may be done regularly throughout the

Substance Abuse

Indiscriminate use of alcohol or drugs such as cocaine, PCP, opiates, and methadone may affect the woman and her fetus/neonate. Alcohol abuse has been associated with fetal alcohol syndrome. Use of addicting drugs may cause the infant to be born addicted or to have serious and permanent problems.

Signs of addiction in the pregnant woman may include dilated or constricted pupils, inflamed nasal mucosa, abscesses, edema or track marks on arms and legs, inappropriate or disoriented behavior, or excessive fatigue. Risks to the fetus include the following (varies somewhat according to substance abuse):

1. *Be alert for* signs of substance abuse. If it is suspected, ask direct questions, beginning with less threatening questions about use of tobacco, caffeine, and alcohol consumption. Then progress to questions about illicit drugs.

(Continued)

63

Table 2–1 Selected Complications during Pregnancy *(continued)*

Condition/Overview	Signs/Symptoms/Risk	Medical Therapy	Nursing Interventions
	neurologic changes, including marked irritability, poor interactive behavior, poor consolability, seizures, and so forth.	pregnancy for women who are known or suspected substance abusers.	2. Provide information about the possible effects of substance abuse on the fetus.
Multiple Gestation Morbidity and mortality rates increase significantly in pregnancies with multiple fetuses. Dizygotic, or fraternal, twins (resulting from two ova) are more common. Incidence of fraternal twins is affected by heredity, race, maternal age and parity, and fertility drugs. Monozygotic, or identical, twins (resulting from one ovum) are not as common. Incidence is not influenced by external factors other than infertility	Fetal risk is significantly higher. The perinatal mortality rate is higher, and there is an increased risk of preterm labor with the problems associated with prematurity. Multiple gestation increases the incidence of intrauterine growth (IUGR), congenital anomalies, and abnormal presentations. For the mother, a multiple gestation may contribute to more physical discomfort during pregnancy,	Early diagnosis based on history, greater than anticipated uterine size. Ultrasound is crucial. Women are seen every 2 weeks until 28 weeks' gestation and then weekly. Serial ultrasounds are done regularly to assess for IUGR. NST and fetal biophysical profile are done at least weekly beginning at 28–30 weeks. Bed rest in the lateral position may be suggested as early as 23–26 weeks to prevent preterm labor.	1. Counsel on importance of good nutrition including adequate calories (40–45 kcal/kg/day), calcium (1800–2000 mg/day), and protein (more than 1.5 g/kg). 2. Discuss importance of sufficient rest at home (usually bed rest with BRP) or at least two hours in the morning, afternoon, and evening.

therapy. Higher numbers of fetuses (triplets or quadruplets, for example) may result from either process or a combination (Cunningham, et al., 1997).

such as shortness of breath, backaches, and pedal edema, as well as an increased incidence of PIH, anemia, and placenta previa. Prolonged hospitalization may be necessary, especially with three or more fetuses.

Maternal blood pressure is monitored closely. Preterm labor is managed in the same way as it is for single pregnancy (see earlier discussion in this chapter).

3. If woman is hospitalized, explain importance of complete bed rest (or bed rest with BRP is ordered).

4. Monitor fetal status. This involves isolating each FHR as well as running an electronic fetal monitor strip on each fetus at least q4–8h (depending on agency policy). If possible the strips will be run at the same time using two (or three) monitors. This becomes more difficult with quadruplets.

5. Monitor for signs of complications such as PIH or preterm labor.

References

American College of Obstetricians and Gynecologists (ACOG). (1999). *Scheduled cesarean delivery and the prevention of vertical transmission of HIV infection* (ACOG Committee Opinion 219). Washington, DC: Author.

American Diabetes Association (ADA). (2000a). Position statement: Gestational diabetes mellitus. *Diabetes Care, 23*(Suppl. 1), S77–S79.

American Diabetes Association (ADA). (2000b). Position statement: Preconception care of women with diabetes. *Diabetes Care, 23*(Suppl. 1), S65–S68.

Centers for Disease Control and Prevention (CDC). (1998). 1998 guidelines for the treatment of sexually transmitted disease. *Mortality and Morbidity Weekly Report, 47* (RR–1), 1–116.

Chez, R. A. (1999). Prevention of preterm birth: Putting three new tools into practice. *Contemporary OB/GYN, 44*(6), 53–78.

Creasy, R. K., & Iams, J. D. (1999). Preterm labor and delivery. In R. K. Creasy & R. Resnick (Eds.), *Maternal-fetal medicine* (4th ed., pp. 498–531). Philadelphia: Saunders.

Cunningham, F. G., MacDonald, P. C., Gant, N. F., Leveno, K. J., Gilstrap, L. C., Hankins, G. C. V., & Clark, L. L. (1997). *Williams obstetrics* (20th ed.). Stamford, CT: Appleton & Lange.

Curet, L. B. (2000). Obstetric management of diabetes mellitus in pregnancy. In J. J. Sciarra (Ed.), *Maternal and fetal medicine* (Vol. 3, pp. 1–10).

Landon, M. B. (2000). Obstetric management of pregnancies complicated by diabetes mellitus. *Clinical Obstetrics and Gynecology, 43*(1), 65–74.

Mandeville, I., & Troiano, N. (1992). *High-risk intrapartum nursing*. Philadelphia: Lippincott.

Spellacy, W. N. (1999). Diabetes mellitus and pregnancy. In J. R. Scott et al. (Eds.), *Danforth's obstetrics and gynecology* (8th ed., pp. 301–308). Philadelphia: Lippincott Williams & Wilkins.

Chapter 3

The Intrapartal Client

Labor and birth progresses through four stages. A first-time laboring woman (nullipara) *averages* 13 hours (11 hours in first stage and 2 hours of pushing in second stage). A multipara *averages* about 8 hours (7¼ hours in first stage and 1 hour pushing in second stage). See Table 3–1 for definitions of each stage of labor.

Nursing Care during Admission

Admission is a critical time for data collection that will aid in the formation of nursing care for the laboring family.

- Orient laboring woman and her support team to the room and the equipment.
- Instruct woman to change into hospital gown.
- Obtain a urine specimen if membranes are intact and woman is not bleeding.
- Assess uterine activity, fetal status, and status of membranes.
- Assess temperature, blood pressure, pulse, and respirations.
- Complete admission forms and consent forms.
- Review prenatal record for history of pregnancy (present and past), preexisting medical problems, estimated date of

Table 3–1 Stages of Labor and Birth

Stage	Begins	Ends
First	Beginning of cervical dilatation	Complete dilatation
Second	Complete dilatation	Birth of the baby
Third	Birth of the baby	Birth of the placenta
Fourth	Birth of the placenta	1–4 hours past birth

birth (EDB), risk factors, blood type and Rh, allergies, medications, and history of substance abuse.

• Discuss the method of desired pain management.

• Determine the desired role of the support team.

• Notify physician or certified nurse-midwife of woman's labor status.

• See Table 3–2 for deviations from normal labor process that require immediate interventions.

Sample Admission Nurse's Charting

Grav I Para 0 EDB 7/13. 40 wks gestation. Admitted ambulatory to BR1 in labor. Contractions q3min, 50 sec duration of mod qual. Memb intact. Cervix 5 cm, 80% effaced, soft and anterior. Small amount blood-tinged mucus present. Vertex presentation at 0 station. FHR 140 by external fetal monitoring. No increase or decrease in FHR noted during or following UC. Average variability. Maternal temp 98.6°F, pulse 78, resp 18, BP 120/74. Adm UA obtained and to lab. Support person with pt and to remain through birth. Pt. oriented to room. P. Gomez, RNC

Assessment of Uterine Activity during Labor

• Uterine activity can be assessed by either palpation or electronic monitoring.

• Assess for frequency, duration, and intensity. (*Note:* Assess a minimum of three consecutive contractions when evaluating uterine activity.)

• See Table 3–3 for contraction and labor progress characteristics.

1. **Frequency** is timed from the beginning of a contraction (when the uterus first begins to tighten) to the beginning of the next contraction. Frequency is recorded in minutes.

2. **Duration** is timed from the beginning of a contraction (when the uterus first begins to tighten) to the end of

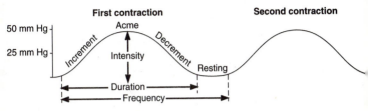

Figure 3–1   Characteristics of uterine contractions.

that same contraction (when the uterus fully relaxes). Duration is recorded in seconds.

3. **Intensity** refers to the strength of a contraction during the acme. It is evaluated by estimating the indentability of the fundus at the acme of the contraction when using palpation as method of evaluation or by the use of an intrauterine pressure catheter (IUPC). Intensity is recorded as mild, moderate, or strong when palpating contraction and in millimeters of mercury when using an IUPC.

- See Figure 3–1 for characteristics of uterine contractions.

Palpating Uterine Contractions

- With the woman's gown over her abdomen but blanket pulled down, place palmer surface of fingertips on the fundal area of the uterus.
- Assess for frequency, duration, and intensity.
  1. Mild intensity: At the acme of the contraction the fingertips can easily indent the abdomen.
  2. Moderate intensity: At the acme of the contraction the fingertips can slightly indent the abdomen.
  3. Strong: At the acme of the contraction the fingertips cannot indent the abdomen.

Record assessment findings in chart.

Table 3–2 Deviations from Normal Labor Process Requiring Immediate Intervention

Finding	Immediate Action	Finding	Immediate Action
Woman admitted with unusual vaginal bleeding or history of painless vaginal bleeding	1. Do not perform vaginal examination. 2. Assess FHR. 3. Evaluate amount of blood loss. 4. Evaluate labor pattern. 5. Notify physician/CNM immediately.	Prolapse of umbilical cord	1. Relieve pressure on cord manually. 2. Continuously monitor FHR; watch for changes in FHR pattern. 3. Notify physician/CNM. 4. Assist woman into knee-chest position. 5. Administer oxygen. 6. Direct another person to prepare for immediate cesarean section. 7. Watch for decreasing baseline, loss of variability, presence of late or variable decelerations.
Presence of greenish or brownish amniotic fluid	1. Continuously monitor FHR. 2. Evaluate dilatation status of cervix and determine whether umbilical cord is prolapsed. 3. Evaluate presentation (vertex or breech). 4. Maintain woman on complete bed rest on left side. 5. Notify physician/CNM immediately. 6. Note color and consistency of amniotic fluid.		

| Absence of FHR and fetal movement | 1. Notify physician/CNM.
2. Provide truthful information and emotional support to laboring couple.
3. Remain with the couple.
4. Prepare for diagnostic ultrasound exam. |
| Woman admitted in advanced labor; birth imminent | 1. Prepare for immediate birth.
2. Obtain critical information:
  a. EDB
  b. History of bleeding problems
  c. History of medical or obstetrical problems
  d. Past and or present use/abuse of prescription/OTC/illicit drugs
  e. Problems with this pregnancy
  f. FHR and maternal vital signs if possible
  g. Whether membranes are ruptured and how long since rupture
  h. Blood type and Rh
3. Direct another person to contact CNM/physician; do not leave woman alone.
4. Provide support to couple.
5. Put on gloves. |

Table 3–3 Contraction and Labor Progress Characteristics

Contraction Characteristics	
Latent phase	Every 10–20 min × 15–20 sec; mild, progressing to
	Every 5–7 min × 30–40 sec; moderate
Active phase	Every 2–3 min × 60 sec; moderate to strong
Transition phase	Every 2 min × 60–75 sec; strong
Labor Progress Characteristics	
Primipara	1.2 cm/h dilatation
	1 cm/h descent
	<2 h in second stage (3 h with epidural)
Multipara	1.5 cm/h dilatation
	2 cm/h descent
	<1 h in second stage (2 h with epidural)

Assessment by External Electronic Uterine Monitoring

- With the woman's gown up and blanket down, place the tocodynamometer (toco) against the fundal area of the uterus. The toco is held into place with elastic belts.
- Assess for frequency and duration.
- Uterine contraction intensity cannot be evaluated accurately with external electronic monitoring.
- Record assessment findings in chart.

Assessment by Intrauterine Pressure Catheter (IUPC)

- Membranes must be ruptured prior to placement of the IUPC.
- Explain procedure to woman and her labor support team.
- Have IUPC in room ready for placement.
- Certified nurse-midwife or physician inserts IUPC into uterine cavity.
- IUPC is connected to electronic monitor.

- Frequency, duration, and intensity are recorded on the monitor strip.
- Normal resting pressure is below 20 mm Hg.
- During the acme the intensity ranges from
  1. 25 to 40 mm Hg in the latent phase.
  2. 50 to 70 mm Hg in the active phase.
  3. 70 to 90 mm Hg in the transition phase.
  4. 70 to 100 mm Hg in the second stage while the woman is pushing.

Frequency of Assessments for Low-Risk Mother

- Latent phase: Every 30 minutes.
- Active phase: Every 30 minutes.
- Transition: Every 15 to 30 minutes.
- Second stage: Continuously.

Assessment of Cervical Changes

Cervical assessment evaluates cervical dilatation and efface-ment and position of the cervix. These data are obtained by in-trapartal vaginal examination (Figure 3–2). See Procedure: Performing Intrapartal Vaginal Examination, page 310.

Dilatation   Enlargement of the external cervical os from 0 to 10 cm.

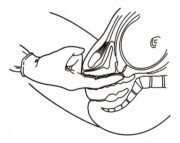

Figure 3–2   Determination of cervical dilatation.

Effacement　　　The drawing up of the internal os and cervical canal into the uterine side wall. This is measured in percentages: 0% indicates no effacement, and 100% indicates full effacement. In nulliparas, effacement usually precedes dilatation.

Assessment of Amniotic Fluid Membranes

It is important to determine whether amniotic membranes are intact or ruptured. The woman's risk for ascending bacterial infection is increased after the membranes have ruptured.

Membranes Ruptured Prior to Admission to Labor Unit

- Ask woman when the membranes ruptured (when she felt a gush of fluid from her vagina).
- Note the color (should be colorless), odor (should be odorless), and amount (small, moderate, or large) of fluid.
- To confirm the rupture of membranes the nurse can check with nitrazine paper or by use of the ferning test.
- **Nitrazine paper test:**
  1. Explain procedure to woman and position for intrapartal exam.
  2. Items needed: sterile glove and nitrazine paper.
  3. With a sterile, unlubricated, gloved hand, insert nitrazine into cervical area and remove it.
  4. Nitrazine paper is sensitive to pH and will turn blue when exposed to amniotic fluid.
  5. Discuss findings with woman.
- **Ferning test:**
  1. Explain procedure to woman and position for intrapartal exam.
  2. Items needed: sterile glove, lubricant, Q-Tip, and slide.
  3. With a sterile gloved hand obtain a swabbed specimen of vaginal fluid.

4. Apply fluid to a microscopic slide and let dry. Then observe slide under magnification.

5. A frondlike pattern will appear with crystallization of amniotic fluid.

6. Discuss findings with woman.

- Assess fetal status via auscultation or electronic fetal monitoring (see discussion in the next section).
- Assess for prolapsed cord via intrapartal exam.
- Chart findings, including date and time of rupture, color of fluid, odor of fluid, amount of fluid, and fetal status.

Membranes Rupture after Admission to Labor Unit

- Note the time of rupture, the color of the fluid, the odor, and the amount.
- Assess FHR via auscultation or electronic fetal monitoring.
- There is an increased risk of a prolapsed umbilical cord if the membranes rupture prior to engagement of the presenting part. Assess for prolapsed cord via intrapartal exam: Can you feel the cord around the cervical area?
- Chart findings that include time of rupture, color of fluid, odor of fluid, amount of fluid, and fetal status.

Assessment of Fetus

Fetal Heart Rate

Fetal heart rate can be assessed with the use of a fetoscope, Doppler, tocotransducer, or fetal scalp electrode.

- **Baseline rate:** Refers to the range of FHR observed between contractions during a 10-minute period of monitoring. The range does not include the rate present during decelerations. Normal range is 120–160 bpm.
- **Baseline changes:** Defined in terms of 10-minute periods of time. Changes include tachycardia, bradycardia, and variability of heart rate.

- **Tachycardia:** FHR above 160 bpm continuing for 10 minutes or longer.
- **Bradycardia:** FHR less than 110 bpm continuing for 10 minutes or longer.
- **Periodic changes:** Refers to the presence of acceleration and deceleration.
- Other characteristics of electronic fetal monitoring (EFM) tracings are presented in Table 3–4.

Assessment Using Fetoscope or Doppler

See Procedure: Auscultating Fetal Heart Rate, page 297.

Assessment Using External Electronic Fetal Monitor

See Procedure: Electronic Fetal Monitoring, page 302.

Evaluation of Fetal Monitor Tracing

Evaluation of monitor tracing includes uterine activity and fetal heart rate. A 10-minute strip is needed to evaluate uterine activity and fetal heart rate. See Figure 3–3.
- Uterine activity:
  1. Determine uterine resting tone.
  2. Determine frequency, duration, and intensity of the contractions.
- Fetal heart rate:
  1. Determine baseline rate.
  2. Assess for bradycardia or tachycardia.
- Determine variability: Is it marked, average, minimal, or absent? Assess for accelerations, decelerations, and sinusoidal pattern.
- Assess for periodic changes (see following discussion).
- See Table 3–4 for characteristics of FHR tracings.

Types of Periodic Changes
- **Accelerations:** Transient increases in FHR of 15 bpm above baseline for 15 seconds. They are usually caused by fetal movement. These are signs of fetal well-being.

Table 3-4 Characteristics of FHR Tracings

Example	Characteristic	Nursing Intervention
(tracing, scale 3–18, 60–210, ←1 minute→) **Increased LTV; STV present**	*Variability* Defined as long term or short term. Caused by interplay of sympathetic and parasympathetic nervous system. Long-term variability (LTV) classification: Decreased/minimal: 0–5 bpm Moderate/average: 6–25 bpm Marked (saltatory): >25 bpm	Maximize uteroplacental perfusion by positioning woman on left side. Document findings; report status to certified nurse-midwife (CNM) or physician. Correct maternal hypotension by turning woman to side-lying position, increasing rate of intravenous infusion. For the most part, there are no specific interventions.
(tracing) **Average LTV; STV absent**	Short-term variability (STV) is classified as present or absent. *Nonperiodic Accelerations* An increase of FHR that lasts for a few seconds. Occurs with fetal movement. Is basis of nonstress test (NST).	(tracing) FHR / UC / **A** accelerations that occur spontaneously
(tracing) **Absent LTV; STV present**		

Table 3–4 Characteristics of FHR Tracings *(continued)*

Example	Characteristic	Nursing Intervention
(FHR scale 210, 180, 150, 120, 90, 60; 18, 15, 12, 9, 6, 3)	*Deceleration*	
	Periodic decrease in FHR from the normal baseline.	No specific intervention needed.
	Classified as early, late, or variable.	Monitor for changes in FHR pattern.
Absent LTV; STV absent	*Early Deceleration (Periodic)*	Evaluate for possible cephalopelvic disproportion (CPD) if occurs in early labor.
(scale 21, 18, 15, 12, 9, 6, 3, 0 and 240, 210, 180, 120, 90, 60, 30; labels "Onset of deceleration" and "End of deceleration")	Due to pressure on the fetal head as it progresses down the birth canal.	
	Characteristics:	
	Resembles upside-down shape of uterine contraction.	
	Occurs at or just before the beginning of contraction and ends as contraction ends.	
(scale 500, 375, 250, 125, 0 and 100, 75, 50, 25, 0; mm Hg)	Nadir (lowest point) occurs at peak of contraction and is within normal FHR range.	
	Is considered a normal variation.	

Late Deceleration (Periodic)

Due to uteroplacental insufficiency as the result of decreased blood flow and oxygen transfer to the fetus during contractions.

Characteristics:

Smooth, uniform shape that inversely mirrors contraction.

Begins at or within seconds after the peak of the contraction.

Lasts past end of contraction.

Tends to occur with every contraction; persistent and consistent.

Usually occurs within normal FHR range.

In some situations, changing maternal position, providing IV hydration, and decreasing contraction frequency decrease late decelerations.

Variable Deceleration (Nonperiodic)

Due to umbilical cord compression, which decreases the amount of blood flow (therefore oxygen supply) to the fetus.

Turn woman to left side-lying position.

Report findings to physician/CNM and document findings.

Provide explanation to woman and partner.

Monitor for further FHR changes.

Maintain good hydration with IV fluids.

Discontinue oxytocin if it is being administered.

Administer oxygen by face mask at 7–10 L/min.

Monitor maternal BP, P for signs of hypotension.

Assist with preparation for cesarean birth if required.

Document findings.

Report status to certified nurse-midwife/physician.

(Continued)

240
210
180
150
120
90
60
30

21
18
15
12
9
6- End of deceleration
3
0
Onset of deceleration

100
75
50
25
0

500
375
250
125
0

mm Hg

Table 3–4 Characteristics of FHR Tracings *(continued)*

Example	Characteristic	Nursing Intervention
	Characteristics: Varies in onset, occurrence, and waveform. Usually falls outside the normal FHR range. Is acute in onset.	Change maternal position to one on which FHR pattern is most improved. Correct maternal hypotension. Assist with preparation for cesarean birth if required. Provide explanation to woman and partner. Discontinue oxytocin if it is being administered and there are severe variables. Oxytocin may be continued if mild or moderate decelerations are present. Perform vaginal examination to assess for prolapsed cord or change in labor progress. Monitor FHR continuously to assess current status and for further changes in FHR pattern.

Source: Association of Women's Health, Obstetrical, and Neonatal Nurses (AWHONN), 1997.

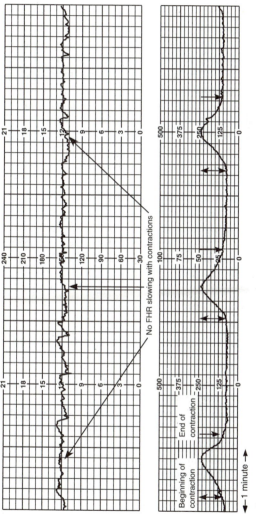

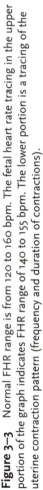

Figure 3–3   Normal FHR range is from 120 to 160 bpm. The fetal heart rate tracing in the upper portion of the graph indicates FHR range of 140 to 155 bpm. The lower portion is a tracing of the uterine contraction pattern (frequency and duration of contractions).

81

- **Early decelerations:** Deceleration that begins with the onset of a contraction and ends before the contraction ends. They are uniform in shape and are due to head compression. Interventions are not needed.
- **Late decelerations:** Decelerations that start after the beginning of the contraction and end after the contraction ends. They are uniform in shape and are due to uteroplacental insufficiency. Interventions are needed.
- **Variable decelerations:** Decelerations that vary in onset, occurrence, and shape. They are due to umbilical cord compression. Interventions are needed.

Classifying the FHR Tracing as Reassuring or Nonreassuring

- **Reassuring pattern:** FHR baseline between 120 and 160 bpm, average variability, acceleration with fetal movement, absence of late or variable deceleration.
- **Nonreasurring pattern:** Late decelerations, absence of variability, prolonged deceleration, bradycardia, variable decelerations associated with decreasing variability, or variable decelerations with slow return of FHR to baseline.

  Note: Nonreassuring pattern may indicate fetal distress, which requires interventions.

Fetal Presentation, Position, and Station

- See Figure 3–4.
- Fetal presentation, position, and station are determined by intrapartal vaginal examination.
- **Presentation:** Refers to the part of the fetus that enters the pelvic passage first. Fetal presentation may be cephalic, breech, or transverse.
- **Position:** Refers to the relationship of a designated landmark on the presenting fetal part to the front, back, or side of the maternal pelvis. Examples of cephalic positions are the following:
  1. OA, occiput anterior.
  2. ROA, right occiput anterior.

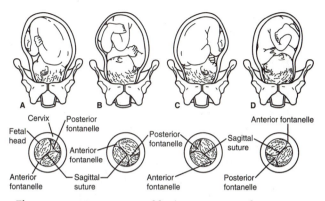

Figure 3-4   Assessment of fetal position. **A,** Left occiput anterior (LOA). The posterior fontanelle (triangle shaped) is in the upper left quadrant of the maternal pelvis. **B,** Left occiput posterior (LOP). The posterior fontanelle is in the lower left quadrant of the maternal pelvis. **C,** Right occiput anterior (ROA). The posterior fontanelle is in the upper right quadrant of the maternal pelvis. **D,** Right occiput posterior (ROP). The posterior fontanelle is in the lower right quadrant of the maternal pelvis.

3. LOA, left occiput anterior.
4. LOT, left occiput transverse.
5. OP, occiput posterior.
6. LOP, left occiput posterior.
7. ROP, right occiput posterior.
8. ROA, right occiput anterior.

- **Station:** Refers to the relationship of the presenting part to the ischial spines. It measures fetal descent.

Psychosocial Considerations

Assessment of the woman's emotional state, her coping methods, and her support system will provide useful information for the admission process and later in the labor.

- Assessment data:
  1. Determine type of prenatal education program the woman has completed.
  2. Determine her hopes or plans for the labor and birth experience.
  3. Determine plans she has made with her certified nurse-midwife or physician.
  4. Determine her informational needs.
  5. Determine the roles of her support team.
  6. Assess for evidence of support between the woman and her partner and/or support team.
  7. Assess her past labor and birth experiences.
  8. Assess for cultural needs during labor and birth.
  9. Determine her desired method of pain management.

Assessing for Safety and Abuse Issues

- Physical and/or mental abuse affects 25% to 30% of pregnant women (McFarland & Gondolf, 1998).
- Interview woman alone when assessing safety and abuse issues to ensure that she can freely answer questions.
- Questions to ask include the following:
  1. Have you ever been emotionally or physically abused by your partner or someone important to you?
  2. Within the last year, have you been hit, slapped, kicked, or otherwise physically hurt by someone? If yes, by whom? Total number of times?
  3. Since you've been pregnant, were you hit, slapped, kicked, or otherwise physically hurt by someone? If yes, by whom? Total number of times?
  4. Within the last year has anyone forced you to engage in sexual activities? If yes, who? Total number of times?
  5. Are you afraid of your partner or anyone you mentioned earlier?

Critical Nursing Assessments during Labor

During the first stage of labor the nurse assesses

- Uterine contractions.
- Fetal status.
- Status of membranes and amniotic fluid.
- Maternal temperature, blood pressure, pulse, and respirations.
- Maternal comfort level and need for pain management assistance.
- Needs of support team.

See Table 3–5 for nursing assessment during labor and birth.

Critical Nursing Interventions during Labor

During labor, the nursing support measures vary depending on the progress of labor and the wishes of the laboring woman or couple. Table 3–6 summarizes the major characteristics of labor and birth and presents nursing interventions that may be used in each stage of labor.

Pain Management during Labor

- Pain during the first stage of labor is due to cervical stretching.
- Pain during the second stage of labor is due to stretching of the vagina and perineum.
- A variety of methods and techniques can be used for labor pain management.
- Nonpharmacologic methods include visualization, relaxation techniques, breathing patterns, and touch.

Visualization Method

- Direct the woman to visualize a place where she has a pleasant memory or feeling: "Think of a place where you

Table 3–5 Nursing Assessments during Labor and Birth

Stage	Maternal Assessments	Fetal Assessments
First Stage Latent phase	Blood pressure, pulse, respirations q1h if in normal range. Temperature q4h unless over 37.5°C (99.6°F) or membranes ruptured, then q1h. Uterine contractions q30min.	FHR q60min for low-risk women and q30min for high-risk women, if normal characteristics present (average variability, baseline in the 120–160 beats/minute range, without late or variable decelerations.
Active phase	BP, P, R q1h if in normal range. Uterine contractions q30min.	Note fetal activity. If EFM in place, assess for reactive NST.
Transition	BP, P, R q30min.	FHR q30min for low-risk women and q15min for high-risk women, if normal characteristics are present. FHR q30min for low-risk women and q15min for high-risk women.
Second Stage	BP, P, R q5–15min. Uterine contractions palpated with each contraction or continuously.	FHR q15min for low-risk women and q5min for high-risk women.

Source: Nurses Association of American College of Obstetricians and Gynecologists (NAACOG), 1990.

Table 3–6 Normal Progress, Psychologic Characteristics, and Nursing Support during First and Second Stages of Labor

Stage/ Phase	Cervical Dilatation	Uterine Contractions	Woman's Response	Nursing Support Measures
Stage 1 Latent phase	1–3 cm	Every 10–20 min, 15–30 sec duration. Mild intensity progressing to moderate.	Usually happy, talkative, and eager to be in labor. Exhibits need for independence by taking care of own bodily needs and seeking information.	Establish rapport on admission and continue to build during care. Assess information base and learning needs. Be available to consult regarding breathing technique if needed; teach breathing technique if needed and in early labor. Orient family to room, equipment, monitors, and procedures. Encourage woman and partner to participate in care as desired. Provide needed information. Assist woman into position of comfort (nonsupine position); encourage frequent change of position; and encourage ambulation during early labor. Offer fluids/ice chips. Keep couple informed of progress. Encourage woman to void every 1 to 2 hours. Assess need for and interest in using visualization to enhance relaxation and teach if appropriate.

(Continued)

Table 3–6 Normal Progress, Psychologic Characteristics, and Nursing Support during First and Second Stages of Labor *(continued)*

Stage/ Phase	Cervical Dilatation	Uterine Contractions	Woman's Response	Nursing Support Measures
Active phase	4–7 cm	Every 2–3 min, 40–60 sec duration. Moderate intensity.	May experience feelings of helplessness; exhibits increased fatigue and may begin to feel restless and anxious as contractions become stronger; expresses fear of abandonment. Becomes more dependent as she is less able to meet her needs.	Observe response to contractions. Encourage woman to maintain breathing patterns; provide quiet environment to reduce external stimuli. Provide reassurance, encouragement, support; keep couple informed of progress. Promote comfort by giving back rubs, sacral pressure, cool cloth on forehead, assistance with position changes, support with pillows, effleurage. Provide ice chips, ointment for dry mouth and lips. Encourage to void every 1 to 2 hours. Offer shower/Jacuzzi/warm bath if available.
Transition	8–10 cm	Every 2–3 min, 60–75 sec duration. Strong intensity.	Tires and may exhibit increased restlessness and irritability; may feel she cannot keep up with labor process and is out of control. Physical discomforts. Fear of being left alone. May fear tearing open or splitting apart with contractions.	Encourage woman to rest between contractions; if she sleeps between contractions, wake her at beginning of contraction so she can begin breathing pattern (increases feeling of control). Provide support, encouragement, and praise for efforts. Keep couple informed of progress; encourage continued participation of support persons. Promote comfort as noted earlier but

			recognize many women do not want to be touched when in transition. Provide privacy. Provide ice chips, ointment for lips. Encourage to void every 1 to 2 hours.
			If she has difficulty focusing, cup your hands close to her face and place your face close to hers. Talk her through the contraction. Have her breathe with you. Stay with her.
Stage 2	Complete	Every 2 minutes. 60–75 seconds, strong.	May feel out of control, helpless, panicky, exhausted, exhilarated.	Assist woman in pushing efforts. Encourage woman to assume position of comfort. She may be most comfortable in a sitting position on a toilet, leaning over a birthing bar, on hands and knees, or perhaps on her side. Some women like to sit in high Fowler's, to have support behind their shoulders, and to have someone hold their legs up and flexed while they push. Provide encouragement and praise for efforts. Keep couple informed of progress. Provide ice chips and cool cloth for forehead. Maintain privacy as woman desires.

have been that has pleasant memories and feelings around it, a place that was relaxing, where all your stress disappeared."

- Ask the woman to take in a breath and remember the smells around the place. If it was outside, instruct her to feel the warmth of the sun or the way the breeze felt on her face.
- Instruct her to mentally sit in that place again and let all her tension and tiredness leave her body as she feels the warmth and breezes.
- Give the woman a few moments to think about her special place. Ask if she would like to share information about the setting.
- After the woman has a visualization set up, suggest thinking about it during contractions as a means of increasing relaxation and focusing concentration.
- As each contraction begins, instruct her to think about this special place for a moment and let her body relax.
- Instruct her to keep a picture of her place in her mind as she breathes with the contraction.
- When the contraction is over, instruct her to let her body stay relaxed and to feel the comfort of the room and support of those around her.

Relaxation Techniques

- Assist the woman into a comfortable position (mid-Fowler's with arms supported by pillows, or side-lying with pillow between knees and pillows to support arms, or in a reclining or rocking chair).
- Teach her to breathe slowly and easily and to close her eyes and to let her body sink into the bed (or chair).
- Adjust her position so that each part of her body is supported and comfortable.
- Instruct her to maintain her breathing and try to keep her mind clear.
- Assist her to focus by instructing her to think of the number 1 as she inhales, and the number 2 as she exhales.

- Explain to her that each time her mind begins to drift away to quietly think about the numbers.
- Recommend that she tighten her face, hold it a few seconds, and then release all the tightness. Encourage her to let her tension flow out with her breath.
- A variation of this exercise is to have the woman tighten a body part, hold for a few seconds, and then release it as the coach lightly strokes that body part. Later in labor, gentle stroking of the woman's arms or back will enhance relaxation.

Lamaze Breathing Patterns

- Slow-paced breathing pattern: (Figure 3–5)
    1. This pattern begins and ends with a cleansing breath.
    2. Cleansing breath is inhaled through the nose and exhaled through pursed lips as if cooling a spoonful of hot food.
    3. While inhaling through the nose and exhaling through pursed lips, slow breaths are taken, moving only the chest.
    4. The rate should be approximately six to nine per minute or two breaths in 15 seconds.
    5. The coach or nurse may assist by reminding the woman to take a cleansing breath and then the breaths could be counted out if needed to maintain pacing.
    6. The woman inhales as someone counts "one one thousand, two one thousand, three one thousand,

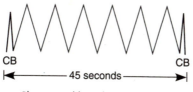

Figure 3–5   Slow-paced breathing.

four one thousand." Exhalation begins and continues through the same count.

- Modified-paced breathing pattern: (Figure 3–6)
  1. This pattern begins and ends with a cleansing breath.
  2. Breaths are then taken in and out silently through the mouth at approximately four breaths in 5 seconds.
  3. The jaw and entire body need to be relaxed.
  4. The rate can be accelerated to 2 to 2½ breaths/second.
  5. The rhythm for the breaths can be counted out as "one and two and one and two and . . ." with the woman exhaling on the numbers and inhaling on "and."

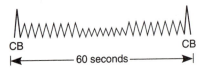

CB　　　　　　　　　　　　　　　　　　CB

|◄———— 60 seconds ————►|

Figure 3–6　Modified-paced breathing.

- Paced breathing pattern: (Figure 3–7)
  1. This pattern begins and ends with a cleansing breath.
  2. All breaths are rhythmical, in and out through the mouth.
  3. Exhalations are accompanied by a "Hee" or "Hoo" sound in a varying pattern, which begins as 3:1 (Hee Hee Hee Hoo) and can change to 2:1 (Hee Hee Hoo) or 1:1 (Hee Hoo) as the intensity of the contraction changes.

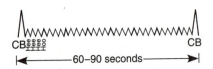

CB　　　　　　　　　　　　　　　　　　CB

|◄———— 60–90 seconds ————►|

Figure 3–7　Paced breathing pattern.

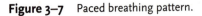

4. The rate should not be more rapid than 2 to 2½ per second.

5. The rhythm of the breaths would match a "one and two and . . ." count.

Therapeutic Touch

- Some women find comfort in being touched during labor.
- Determine if the woman likes being touched.
- Touch or massage a body area of the woman such as the shoulders, arms, hands, legs, feet, or abdomen.
- The touch should be gentle and the massage should be slow and rhythmical.
- Counter sacral pressure or massage may be helpful in reducing back discomfort.

Analgesic Agents for Use during Labor

- A variety of analgesic agents, such as butorphanol tartate (Stadol) or naloxone (Narcan), can be used for labor pain management.
- Analgesics are not given if maternal vital signs are unstable, if the woman is hypotensive, if severe hemorrhage is present, or if the baby is preterm.
- The guidelines for administration are as follows:

  1. Assess woman and her record for history of allergies.
  2. Assess baseline FHR and maternal vital signs prior to administration of analgesic in order to have a comparison if hypotension or FHR changes occur. Record findings on the chart and on EFM strip (if running).
  3. Encourage woman to empty her bladder prior to administration of analgesic to enhance the rest and relaxation from the drug.
  4. Raise side rails to provide safety and explain this precaution to client.
  5. Monitor maternal vital signs and FHR to ensure they remain in a normal range.
  6. Chart analgesic administration and maternal-fetal status on client record and on EFM tracing.

Regional Blocks

- Regional blocks include epidural, spinal-epidural, pudendal, and local infiltration.
- See Table 3–7, which highlights nursing actions during regional blocks.

Continuous Epidural Infusion

Increasing numbers of women are choosing epidurals as their method of labor pain management.

- An epidural relieves pain associated with the first stage by blocking the sensory nerve supply to the uterus.
- An epidural can also relieve pain associated with the second stage of labor.
- Nursing care for women choosing epidurals includes the following:
  1. Explain procedure and equipment.
  2. Assemble equipment needed to administer the epidural.
  3. Begin intravenous infusion with an 18-gauge plastic indwelling catheter.
  4. A bolus of 500–1000 mL is given prior to the administration of the epidural to decrease the risk of hypotension.
  5. Assist woman to the bathroom to void or insert Foley catheter.
  6. Assist woman into a side-lying position at edge of bed or in a sitting position with legs over side of bed.
  7. The labor nurse or partner supports the woman in this position to help ensure that she does not move during the procedure.
  8. The anesthesiologist or certified nurse anesthetist administers the epidural.
  9. An indwelling catheter is placed and taped to the woman's back.
  10. After the epidural is administered and indwelling catheter is taped, the woman is positioned on her side to reduce risk of compression of the ascending vena cava and the descending aorta.

Table 3-7 Summary of Commonly Used Regional Blocks

Type of Block	Area Affected	Use During Labor and Birth	Nursing Actions
Epidural	Vagina, perineum, and uterus	Given in first stage of labor. May be given in second stage if cesarean birth is required.	Assess woman's knowledge regarding the block. Act as advocate to help her obtain further information if needed. Monitor maternal blood pressure to detect the major side effect, which is hypotension. Provide support and comfort.
Spinal-epidural	Vagina, perineum, and uterus	Given in first stage of labor.	Assess woman's knowledge regarding the block. Act as advocate to help her obtain further information. Monitor maternal vital signs, FHR, and uterine contractions. Provide support and comfort.
Pudendal	Perineum and lower vagina	Given in second stage just prior to birth to provide anesthesia for episiotomy or for low forceps delivery.	Assess woman's knowledge regarding the block. Act as advocate to help her obtain further information if needed.
Local infiltration	Perineum	Administered just before birth to provide anesthesia for episiotomy.	Assess woman's knowledge regarding the block. Provide information as needed. Provide comfort and support. Observe perineum for bruising or other discoloration in the recovery period.

- Following the epidural:
  1. Assess the woman's ability to lift her legs and the level of sensation every 30 minutes to monitor effects of the nerve block.
  2. The anesthesia level is too high if the patient reports numbness in her chest, face, or tongue or any breathing difficulties.
  3. Assess for bladder distention if Foley catheter was not inserted.
  4. Monitor FHR, contraction pattern, cervical changes, blood pressure, respirations, and temperature.
- If hypotension occurs:
  1. Increase IV fluid.
  2. Administer oxygen to increase oxygen concentration to the fetus.
  3. Notify the anesthesiologist or certified nurse anesthetist.
  4. If blood pressure is not restored within 1 to 2 minutes administer ephedrine 5 to 10 mg IV, per physician orders.
- If respiratory rate decreases below 14 respirations per minute, naloxone may be given per physician order to counteract the effects of the anesthetic agent. See Drug Guide: Naloxone Hydrochloride (Narcan), page 277.

Nursing Care at the Time of Birth

- During the second stage of labor the nurse assesses
  1. Uterine contractions.
  2. Fetal status.
  3. Maternal blood pressure, pulse, and respirations.
  4. Maternal comfort level and need for support during the pushing phase.
  5. Needs of support team.

See Table 3–5 for nursing assessments during labor and birth.

- Continue encouragement and support to the woman or family.
- Prepare the birthing area when the time of birth approaches.
- Summon the certified nurse-midwife or physician if not already present.
- Continue maternal-fetal assessments as outlined in Table 3–5.
- With support person, assist the woman in her pushing efforts by supporting her legs or shoulders.
- Prepare an instrument table and other equipment.
- Ready oxygen and suction equipment for both mother and newborn if needed.
- Prepare identification bracelets.
- Just prior to the birth, don sterile gloves and cleanse the perineum.

Nursing Care Immediately after the Birth of the Baby

During the third stage of labor the nurse assesses both the mother and the newborn.

Apgar Score

- The Apgar score for the newborn is done at 1 and 5 minutes of age.
- Table 3–8 summarizes the Apgar scoring system.

Physical Assessment of the Newborn

- Initial assessment of the newborn includes the following:
  1. Respirations.
  2. Apical pulse.
  3. Temperature.
  4. Skin color.
  5. Umbilical cord.

Table 3–8 The Apgar Scoring System

	Score		
Sign	**0**	**1**	**2**
Heart rate	Absent	Slow—below 100	Above 100
Respiratory effort	Absent	Slow, irregular	Good crying
Muscle tone	Flaccid	Some flexion of extremities	Active motion
Reflex irritability	None	Grimace	Vigorous cry
Color	Pale blue	Body pink, blue extremities	Completely pink

Source: Apgar, V. (1966, August). The newborn (Apgar) scoring system: Reflections and advice. *Pediatric Clinics of North America, 13,* 645.

    6. Gestational age.

    7. Sole creases.

- See Table 3–9 for initial newborn evaluation.

Maternal Assessment after Birth

- Assess blood pressure and pulse rate.
- Monitor for signs of placental separation:
    1. Uterus becomes globular in shape and firm.
    2. Uterus rises upward in the abdomen.
    3. Umbilical cord lengthens.
    4. A sudden gush of blood.
- Don disposable gloves when handling the newborn.
- Provide warmth for the newborn by drying with warmed, soft blankets, by placing the newborn under a radiant warmer, or by placing the newborn skin to skin with the mother.
- Maintain a clear airway in the newborn by suctioning with the bulb syringe or by using nasopharyngeal suctioning if needed.
- Prevent infection in the newborn by washing hands thoroughly prior to the birth, maintaining asepsis in placing the umbilical cord clamp, and maintaining asepsis if eye prophylaxis is administered in the birthing area.

Table 3–9   Initial Newborn Evaluation

Assess	Normal Findings
Respirations	Rate 30–60 irregular
	No retractions, no grunting
Apical pulse	Rate 120–160 and somewhat irregular
Temperature	Skin temp above 97.8°F (36.5°C)
Skin color	Body pink with bluish extremities
Umbilical cord	Two arteries and one vein
Gestational age	Should be 38–42 weeks to remain with parents for extended time
Sole creases	Sole creases that involve the heel

In general expect scant amount of vernix on upper back, axilla, groin; lanugo only on upper back; ears with incurving of upper two-thirds of pinnae and thin cartilage that springs back from folding; male genitalia—testes palpated in upper or lower scrotum; female genitalia—labia majora larger; clitoris nearly covered.

In the following situations, newborns should generally be stabilized rather than remaining with parents in the birth area for an extended period of time:

- Apgar is less than 8 at 1 minute and less than 9 at 5 minutes, or a baby requires resuscitation measures (other than whiffs of oxygen).
- Respirations are below 30 or above 60, with retractions and/or grunting.
- Apical pulse is below 120 or above 160 with marked irregularities.
- Skin temperature is below 97.8°F (36.5°C).
- Skin color is pale blue, or there is circumoral pallor.
- Baby is less than 38 or more than 42 weeks' gestation.
- Baby is very small or very large for gestational age.
- There are congenital anomalies involving open areas in the skin (meningomyelocele).

- Ensure correct identification of the newborn by placing identification bracelets on the mother and newborn at birth (in some institutions, an identification band is also placed on the support person) and obtaining newborn's footprints and maternal fingerprint on birth record.
- Continue to provide support to the woman and her partner.
- Maintain birth record for the client chart.
- Monitor maternal blood pressure and pulse and signs of placental separation.

- Administer oxytocin as ordered by physician or certified nurse-midwife. The oxytocin may be added to the IV solution if one has already been started, or it may be given intramuscularly (IM) (frequently the ventrogluteal or vastus lateralis site is used).

Nursing Care in the Immediate Recovery Period

Maternal Assessments in the Fourth Stage

- Assessments are done q15min × 4, q30min × 2, q1–2h × 2.
  1. Assess blood pressure and pulse.
  2. Assess the uterine fundus (Figure 3–8). See Procedure: Assessing the Fundus Following Vaginal Birth, page 288.
  3. After removing the peripad or chux, the perineum is observed for swelling, bruising, or lacerations.

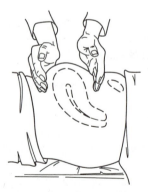

Figure 3–8 Suggested method of palpating the fundus of the uterus during the fourth stage. The left hand is placed just above the symphysis pubis, and gentle downward pressure is exerted. The right hand is cupped around the uterine fundus.

4. Assess the amount of lochia. See Procedure: Evaluating Lochia after Birth, page 305.
5. Assess for bladder distention.

- The nurse can anticipate the findings indicated in Table 3–10.
- The frequent assessments of the immediate recovery cease when
  1. Blood pressure and pulse are stable.
  2. Uterus is firm, in the midline, and below the umbilicus.
  3. Lochia is rubra, moderate in amount, without clots.
  4. Perineum is free from bruising or excessive edema.

Maternal Interventions in the Fourth Stage

- Massage uterus if it becomes soft (boggy).
- Assist mother to the bathroom to void.
- Provide warm blankets if mother experiences postpartum chills.
- Provide fluids and food per physician's order.

Table 3–10   Maternal Adaptations Following Birth

Characteristic	Normal Findings
Blood pressure	Should return to prelabor level
Pulse	Slightly lower than in labor
Uterine fundus	In the midline at the umbilicus or 1–2 finger breadths below the umbilicus
Lochia	Red (rubra), small to moderate amount (from spotting on pads to ¼ to ½ of pad covered in 15 minutes); should not exceed saturation of one pad in first hour
Bladder	Nonpalpable
Perineum	Smooth, pink, without bruising or edema
Emotional state	Wide variation, including excited, exhilarated, smiling, crying, fatigued, verbal, quiet, pensive, and sleepy

- Encourage the mother and partner to hold the infant as they desire.
- Facilitate eye contact with newborn by turning down the lights in the recovery area.
- Explain newborn characteristics.

Newborn Assessments

- Assessments are done q30min × 2, q1h and then q8h if stable.
  1. Assess temperature, pulse, and respirations.
  2. Assess skin color.
  3. Observe for signs of cold stress or hypoglycemia.
  4. If large for gestational age (LGA) or small for gestational age (SGA), assess newborn glucose level via heel stick for capillary blood.

Newborn Interventions

- Maintain newborn temperature by placing a warm blanket over newborn, by placing newborn in skin-to-skin contact with mother, or by placing newborn in a radiant-heated unit.
- If newborn is in a radiant-heated unit, he or she is dried, placed on a warm blanket, and left uncovered.
- Suction nose and mouth with a bulb syringe as needed.
- Apply tetracycline or erythromycin ophthalmic ointment in each eye. See Drug Guide: Erythromycin Ophthalmic Ointment, page 271.
- Give vitamin K 1 mg per physician orders. See Drug Guide: Vitamin K Phytonadione (AquaMephyton), page 280.
- Initiate breastfeeding if desired by mother.

References

Association of Women's Health, Obstetrical, and Neonatal Nurses (AWHONN). (1997). Washington, DC: Author.

McFarland, J., & Parker, B. (1994). Preventing abuse during pregnancy: An assessment and intervention protocol. *Maternal Child Nursing 19*, 321.

Nurses Association of American College of Obstetricians and Gynecologists. (1990, March). *Nursing practice resource: Fetal heart rate auscultation*. Washington, DC: Author.

Chapter 4

The At-Risk Intrapartal Client

Failure to Progress in Labor

- Failure to progress in labor is defined as no progress in cervical dilatation or descent of the presenting part during active labor.
- Failure to progress may be associated with malpresentation (breech, transverse, face, or brow), malposition (occiput posterior), or cephalopelvic disproportion (CPD).
- Failure to progress may also be related to dysfunctional uterine contractions.
- Maternal risks:
  1. Infection secondary to increased number of vaginal examinations to determine status.
  2. Dehydration secondary to inadequate fluid intake.
  3. Exhaustion associated with lengthening of the labor.
- Fetal risks:
  1. Stress secondary to maternal dehydration and subsequent hypotension.
  2. Infection secondary to maternal infection.

Management of Failure to Progress

- Intravenous fluids may be ordered to rehydrate the laboring woman.
- Clinical evaluation to rule out CPD. Physician evaluates cervical dilatation, fetal descent (station), and fetal position.

1. An oxytocin infusion may be started.
2. After 1 hour of adequate uterine contractions, cervical dilatation and fetal station is reevaluated. If progress has been made, labor continues. If no progress has occurred, cesarean birth is indicated.

- If CPD is ruled out and uterine contractions are less than normal in frequency and quality, an oxytocin infusion is started to augment the labor pattern.

Nursing Assessments for Failure to Progress

- Assess fetal vertex for engagement into the maternal pelvis.
- Assess uterine contractions for frequency, duration, and intensity.
- If intensity is less than expected (for this point in labor) and the amount of pain the woman experiences seems out of proportion (feels pain before contraction begins, intense discomfort during contraction, and pain after the contraction is gone), consider the possibility of occiput posterior position.
- Assess cervical dilatation and effacement.
  1. Cervical dilatation usually progresses at 1.5 cm/hour for multiparas and 1.2 cm/hour for primigravidas.
  2. If the cervix becomes edematous and thicker during labor, CPD may be present.
- Assess fetal heart rate (FHR).
- Assess fetal position, presentation, and descent.
- An intrapartal vaginal examination may identify problems such as breech, transverse brow or face presentation, or occiput posterior position.
- Assess for presence of caput (edema of subcutaneous tissues in the top of the fetal head). An enlarging caput may confuse the examiner because it feels like further descent of the fetal head.
- Assess descent of the fetal head by determining station.
- Assess laboring woman for hydration status.
- Assess woman's comfort and coping level.

- Assess support person's level of anxiety, since prolonged labor can be stressful to the support person.

Nursing Diagnoses

- Pain related to inability to relax secondary to labor pattern.
- Risk for ineffective individual coping related to ineffectiveness of breathing techniques to relieve discomfort.

Nursing Interventions for Failure to Progress

- Continuous electronic monitoring of mother and fetus to monitor labor status and fetal status.
- Compare assessment findings to expected norms.
- Assist woman with relaxation and breathing techniques.
- Provide comfort measures such as cool wash cloth to face or back massage.
- Monitor oxytocin infusion if ordered by physician (see discussion later in this chapter).
- Try alternative maternal positions or activity that might facilitate rotation of fetal head or assist with fetal descent. These include standing or walking, sitting on toilet, kneeling, squatting, and taking a warm shower.
- Assist woman to bathroom to void since a full bladder can impede fetal descent.
- Keep the woman and her support team informed of assessment findings and progress.
- Prepare for cesarean birth if indicated.
- Chart assessment findings and nursing and medical interventions.

Sample Nurse's Charting

Contraction every 2½ minutes, 60 sec duration and of strong intensity. Cervical dilatation has remained at 7 cm for 1 hour. FHR BL 140–148 with two accelerations of 15 bpm for 15 sec with fetal movement in the last 20 minutes. Average variability. No decelerations present. Voided 200 mL clear amber urine without difficulty. Taking ice chips at will. Skin turgor and mucous membranes indicate adequate hydration. Breathing with contractions but beginning to cry out at the acme. Dozes between contractions but quickly rouses. Asking "Why is it taking so long? Why am I not making progress?" Partner and family asking to speak with physician regarding treatment plan. Call placed to physician and physician to be here in 5 minutes to see patient. P. Gomez, RNC

Evaluation

1. The woman experiences a more effective labor pattern.
2. The woman has increased comfort and decreased anxiety.

Precipitous Birth

- Precipitous birth is an extremely rapid labor that lasts less than 3 hours from start to finish.
- Maternal risks:
  1. Lacerations of the cervix, vagina, and/or perineum.
  2. Uterine rupture.
  3. Amniotic fluid embolism.
  4. Postpartal hemorrhage.
- Fetal/neonatal risks:
  1. Fetal hypoxia.
  2. Cerebral trauma.

Management of Precipitous Birth

- Close medical monitoring.
- Obtain previous obstetrical history to identify rapid labor.
- Discontinue oxytocin infusion if woman's labor is being induced or augmented.

Nursing Assessments for Precipitous Birth

- Assess previous labor history if the woman is a multipara.
- Assess contraction status. *Be alert for* contractions that are more frequent than every 2 minutes and dilatation that progresses faster than normal (more than 1.5 cm/hour).

- Assess fetal status.
- Assess mother's comfort level.
- Assess mother's coping abilities.

Nursing Diagnoses

- Pain related to accelerated labor pattern.
- Risk for ineffective individual coping related to ineffectiveness of breathing techniques to relieve discomfort.

Nursing Interventions for Precipitous Birth

- Continuous electronic monitoring.
- Notify physician or certified nurse-midwife (CNM) of rapid cervical changes.
- Remain in room to provide support and comfort measures for the woman.
- Instruct woman not to bear down until she is instructed to do so.
- Prepare room for birth.
- Assist with the birth of the baby if the physician or CNM is not present.
  1. Instruct woman to pant with contractions if fetal head is crowning.
  2. Apply gentle pressure against the fetal head to maintain flexion and prevent it from delivering too quickly.
  3. Support the perineum with the other hand and support the descending head between contractions.
  4. Insert two fingers along the back of the fetal neck to check for a nuchal cord. If present, bend the fingers like a fish hook, grasp the cord, and pull it over the baby's head. If the cord cannot be slipped over the head, place two clamps on it and cut between the clamps. Unwind the cord from around the neck.
  5. Suction the fetal nares and mouth with a bulb syringe.

6. While requesting the woman to push gently, exert gentle downward pressure on the head and neck to assist in the birth of the anterior shoulder. Then exert gentle upward pressure to assist with the posterior shoulder. Support the rest of the baby's body as it is born.

7. Place newborn on maternal abdomen and dry the baby with soft warm blankets.

- Check firmness of the uterus. Observe for excessive maternal bleeding.
- Complete client records.

Evaluation

- The woman and her baby are closely monitored during labor and a safe birth occurs.
- The woman states that she feels support and enhanced comfort during labor and birth.

Gestational Age-Related Problems

- See Table 4–1.

Labor Complicated by Malpresentation or Malposition

- See Table 4–2.
- See Figure 4–1 for selected types of fetal malpresentations.

Prolapsed Umbilical Cord

- Prolapsed cord occurs when the umbilical cord precedes the fetus down the birth canal.
- Conditions associated with prolapsed cord:
  1. Breech presentation.
  2. Transverse lie.
  3. Contracted pelvic inlet.
  4. Small fetus.
  5. Extra long cord.

Table 4–1 Babies with Special Needs in Labor and Birth

Type	Implication for Labor	Treatment	Immediate Nursing Support
Postterm	More likely to have decreased amount of amniotic fluid, so variable decelerations are more likely. Meconium may be present in amniotic fluid.	Induction if BPP score decreases, if amniotic fluid volume decreases, or if pregnancy reaches 43 weeks. Amnioinfusion for severe variable decelerations.	Continuous EFM during labor. At birth, assist physician or CNM with visualization of cord and naso-pharyngeal suctioning if fluid is meconium stained.
Preterm	Stress of labor is difficult for baby. Parents are very concerned about baby. Analgesia may be withheld to avoid depressing the fetus/newborn.	Tocolytic therapy to suppress labor. If not successful, forceps may be used to protect fetal head during vaginal birth, or cesarean birth is performed.	Have pediatrician and nursing support available. Provide respiratory support, temperature stabilization, and rapid assessment of newborn.
Multiple gestation	Vertex-vertex presentation is most common, followed by vertex-breech. Increased risk of prolapsed cord and cord entanglement.	Vaginal birth of vertex-vertex presentation may be possible. Other presentations may be possible with guided ultrasound. Continuous EFM of both babies during labor.	For vaginal birth or cesarean birth, double numbers of personnel are required. Provide respiratory support and temperature stabilization.
Macrosomia (weight >4000 g)	CPD is more likely. Dysfunctional labor due to overstretching of uterine muscle fibers.	If CPD present, then cesarean birth performed.	Baby is more likely to develop hypoglycemia. If shoulder dystocia, assess for shoulder movement and crepitus over clavicle.

Table 4-2 Impact of Fetal Malpresentation or Malposition on Birth

Fetal Position	Implication for Labor	Treatment Needed or Anticipated	Nursing Interventions	Impact on Newborn
Occiput posterior	Labor may be longer. Severe back pain may be present.	Forceps or manual rotation at birth may be needed.	Apply sacral pressure. Monitor labor maternal-fetal status. Assist mother into hands-and-knees position and instruct her to do pelvic rock. Alternative position would be to put weight on knees and lean over raised head of bed, change position from side to side, squat, and/or sit on a toilet.	If labor is longer, fetus more likely to experience stress. Head is molded.
Brow presentation (see Figure 4–1)	Labor may be longer.	If CPD is suspected or present, and labor is arrested, then cesarean birth is appropriate.	Monitor labor maternal-fetal status. Provide support measures. Assist with cesarean birth if indicated.	

(Continued)

Table 4–2 Impact of Fetal Malpresentation or Malposition on Birth *(Continued)*

Fetal Position	Implication for Labor	Treatment Needed or Anticipated	Nursing Interventions	Impact on Newborn
Face presentation (see Figure 4–1)	Risks of CPD and prolonged labor are increased.	If no CPD present and chin (mentum) is anterior, vaginal birth may be possible. If chin is posterior a cesarean birth is necessary.	Monitor labor maternal-fetal status. Provide support measures. Assist with cesarean birth if indicated.	May develop facial edema during labor.
Breech (see Figure 4–1)	Labor may be prolonged. Meconium may be expelled in amniotic fluid.	External version may be done at 37–38 weeks and then vaginal birth. If version unsuccessful, cesarean birth is scheduled. Some obstetricians may consider vaginal birth for frank breech.	Monitor labor maternal-fetal status. Monitor for prolapsed cord.	May have edema of throat that compromises breathing. Newborn has increased risk of mortality, intracranial hemorrhage from traumatic birth of head during vaginal birth. Brachial plexus palsy may occur with vaginal birth.

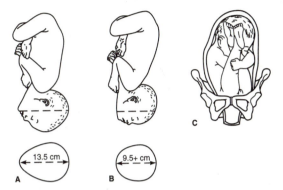

Figure 4–1   Types of malpresentation. **A,** Brow presentation: the largest anterior-posterior diameter presents to the maternal pelvis. **B,** Face presentation: vaginal birth may be possible if the fetal chin is toward the maternal symphysis pubis. **C,** Breech presentation.

6. Low-lying placenta.
7. Hydramnios.
8. Twin gestations.
- Fetal/neonatal risks:
    1. Decreased oxygenation and circulation related to the compressed umbilical cord, with possible fetal distress.

Management of Prolapsed Cord

- Early recognition.
- Once prolapsed cord is identified, an emergency cesarean birth is usually indicated.

Nursing Assessments for Prolapsed Cord

- Assess woman's present pregnancy for conditions associated with prolapsed cord.
- Assess FHR via electronic fetal monitor (EFM), since cord compression is associated with variable decelerations and periodic auscultation may or may not identify a variable deceleration.

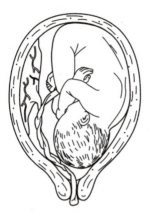

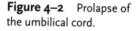
Figure 4–2 Prolapse of the umbilical cord.

- Assess for presence of cord prolapse via intrapartal vaginal exam.
- *Be alert for* the presence of a pulsating, slick cord (see Figure 4–2).

Nursing Diagnoses

- Risk for alteration in gas exchange in the fetus related to decreased blood flow secondary to compression of the umbilical cord.
- Fear related to unknown outcome.

Nursing Interventions for Prolapsed Cord

- Complete an intrapartal vaginal examination to check for prolapse of the cord when variable decelerations are noted on EFM tracing and/or after membranes have ruptured. (See Procedure: Intrapartal Vaginal Examination, page 310.)
- Relieve pressure of the fetal presenting part by leaving the gloved fingers in the vagina and lifting the fetal head off the cord (push fetus up toward the body of the uterus).

- If possible, place woman in knee-chest or Trendelenburg position.
- Maintain the maternal position and pressure on the fetal presenting part until the physician arrives and/or a cesarean birth is accomplished.
- In some instances, an indwelling bladder catheter may be inserted to fill the bladder with warmed normal saline. The filled bladder places upward pressure on the fetal presenting part and relieves pressure on the cord.
- Administer oxygen to the mother by face mask at 7–10 L/minute.
- Call for assistance. Other nurses can assist in the preparation of the woman for emergency cesarean birth.
- Provide information and support to the laboring couple.
- Review the following critical aspects of the care you have provided:
  1. What is the response of the fetal heart rate to the intervention?
  2. Has the rate returned to the 120–160 bpm range?
  3. Is there evidence of variable decelerations on the EFM tracing?
  4. Are the variable decelerations lessening in depth? in number?
  5. Is the position I have asked the woman to assume working? Is FHR improving? Can this position be maintained until a cesarean birth can be accomplished?
  6. Is the baby moving much?
  7. Are accelerations present?
  8. What do I need to protect myself from the woman's bodily fluids? Can a colleague tie a plastic apron around me?

Sample Nurse's Charting

Vaginal exam done to assess dilatation status. Prolapse of the umbilical cord through the cervix and into the vagina. Immediate pressure placed on the fetal vertex. EFM monitor indicates FHR maintained BL of 144–150 from beginning of exam throughout intervention. Variability average. Accelerations of 20 bpm for 15 sec with fetal movement and palpation of fetus. Immediate call placed to Dr. to advise of status. IV of 1000 mL lactated Ringer's started in R wrist after one attempt with 18 ga quikcath. Running at 125 mL/hr. 16Fr indwelling Foley catheter inserted. Abdominal-perineal prep done. To surgery for emergency cesarean section. Continuous pressure placed on fetal vertex through the vagina until birth. Permit signed by husband. P. Gomez, RNC

Hydramnios

- Hydramnios occurs when there is over 2000 mL of amniotic fluid in the amniotic sac.
- The exact cause of hydramnios is unknown; however, it often occurs in cases of major congenital anomalies.
- Maternal risks:
    1. Shortness of breath.
    2. Edema in the lower extremities from compression of the vena cava.
- Fetal/neonatal risks:
    1. Increased risk of mortality due to an increased prevalence of fetal malformations associated with hydramnios.
    2. Increased incidence of preterm birth.
    3. Increased incidence of malpresentation.
    4. Increased incidence of prolapse of the cord.

Management of Hydramnios

- Provide supportive therapy.
- Assess fundal size and monitor growth throughout pregnancy.
- Complete ultrasound examinations to determine presence of anomalies.

- Decrease amount of amniotic fluid. In some instances, an amniocentesis may be done to remove fluid in order to reduce the risk of preterm labor.

Nursing Assessments for Hydramnios

- Assess woman's history for other associated problems such as diabetes, Rh sensitization, fetal malformations, or multiple gestation.
- Assess FHR. It may be more difficult to auscultate the FHR because of the increased amount of fluid. Placement of the EFM may also be more difficult because of the size of the maternal abdomen.
- *Be alert for* the presence of variable decelerations that may indicate prolapse of the cord.
- Assess maternal blood pressure (BP) for hypotension related to compression of the vena cava.
- Assess respiratory rate since weight of the uterus can compromise maternal circulation.
- Assess for fetal malpresentation-malposition by intrapartal vaginal examination of the presenting part.

Nursing Diagnoses

- Risk for impaired gas exchange related to pressure on the diaphragm secondary to hydramnios.
- Fear related to unknown outcome of the pregnancy.

Nursing Interventions for Hydramnios

- Position woman on her left or right side.
- Monitor maternal and fetal status frequently. (See Table 3–5, on page 86.)
- Because of increased incidence of fetal problems, continuous EFM may be warranted.
- Monitor amount of amniotic fluid lost and characteristics of fluid.
- *Be alert for* presence of meconium in the fluid, which may be associated with fetal stress or distress.

Evaluation

- Maternal and fetal status remains stable, with BP, pulse, respirations, and FHR in normal ranges.
- Woman reports that her questions have been answered and her fears have been addressed.

Oligohydramnios

- Oligohydramnios occurs when the amount of amniotic fluid is severely reduced and concentrated.
- The exact cause is unknown; however, it is found in cases of postmaturity, with intrauterine growth restriction (IUGR) secondary to placental insufficiency, and in fetal conditions associated with renal and urinary malfunction.
- Maternal risks:
  1. Dysfunctional labor.
- Fetal risks:
  1. Fetal hypoxia associated with compression of the umbilical cord because the umbilical cord has less fluid to float in.
  2. Increased risk of pulmonary hypoplasia if oligohydramnios has been present throughout the gestation.

Management of Oligohydramnios

- Oligohydramnios is usually identified by serial ultrasound examinations during pregnancy.
- Amnioinfusion (infusion of warmed saline solution) may be done during labor to decrease the risk of cord compression.
- Monitor fetus with biophysical profiles.
- Monitor fetal status.

Nursing Assessments for Oligohydramnios

- Assess the results of any prenatal testing that indicates decreased amniotic fluid volume:
  1. Ultrasound exam with notations of decreased volume.

2. Biophysical profile (BPP) score that is decreased because of diminished amniotic fluid volume.

- Assess FHR:
  1. *Be alert for* variable decelerations.
  2. If membranes rupture, *note* color and amount of fluid.
- Assess for the presence of meconium.

Nursing Diagnoses

- Risk for impaired gas exchange related to pressure on the umbilical cord secondary to decreased amniotic fluid.
- Fear related to unknown outcome of pregnancy.

Nursing Interventions for Oligohydramnios

- Monitor maternal status on a frequent basis:
  1. Watch for hypotension.
  2. Assess for anxiety and tension.
- Monitor fetal status on a frequent basis for signs of decreased placental-fetal profusion. *Be alert for* presence of variable decelerations and decreased variability.
- Encourage woman to maintain side-lying position while in bed.
- Assist with amnioinfusion if done.

Evaluation

- The woman and her partner state that they understand the condition, the need for monitoring, and possible associated problems.
- The woman gives birth to a healthy newborn.

Amniotic Fluid Embolism

- An amniotic fluid embolism is a catastrophic event that occurs when a small amount of amniotic fluid enters the maternal blood stream. The amniotic fluid moves through the maternal circulation, through the right atrium and ventricle, and then into the pulmonary circulation.

- Maternal mortality rate is approximately 70% (Cunningham et al., 1997).
- Symptoms may include the following:
    1. Sudden respiratory distress.
    2. Tachycardia.
    3. Circulatory collapse.
    4. Acute hemorrhage.
    5. Cor pulmonale.
    6. Hypotension.
    7. Shock.
    8. Coma.
- Fetal hypoxia or anoxia occurs as the mother experiences respiratory difficulty or respiratory arrest.

Management of Pulmonary Embolism

- Emergency support measures, which may include intubation, are instituted.
- Immediate intensive care to support circulatory and respiratory systems is required.
- Oxygen is administered by mask or positive pressure.
- Intravenous (IV) therapy is begun.
- Central hemodynamic monitoring lines are necessary to monitor pressures and make treatment decisions.
- Dopamine may be required to maintain maternal blood pressure.
- Coagulation studies are completed to monitor the development of disseminated intravascular coagulation (DIC) and to monitor treatment.
- Continuous EFM is necessary to monitor fetal status (Cunningham et al., 1997).

Nursing Assessments for Pulmonary Embolism

- Assess for associated factors such as multiparity, hydramnios, tumultuous labor (contractions with frequency of less than 2 minutes and strong intensity).

Tumultuous labor may occur naturally or may be associated with intravenous oxytocin administration.

- Assess maternal vital signs.
- *Be alert for* signs of respiratory distress or any statement from the mother that she is experiencing difficulty breathing.
- Assess FHR for rate, variability, and presence of decelerations.
- Assess for hemorrhage and signs of shock.

Nursing Diagnoses

- Risk for impaired gas exchange related to cardiopulmonary collapse.
- Fear related to risk of death secondary to pulmonary embolism.

Nursing Interventions for Pulmonary Embolism

- Continuously monitor and evaluate maternal-fetal status.
- If respiratory difficulties occur
  1. Provide oxygen.
  2. Call for emergency assistance. Provide respiratory and cardiac support until assistance arrives.
  3. Start one or two peripheral IV lines.
  4. Prepare for administration of whole blood.
  5. Prepare for insertion of central venous pressure (CVP) line.
  6. Monitor fluid intake.
  7. Assist with emergency measures.
  8. Have one nurse *note* the type and administration time of all medications.
- Complete client records. Nurses' notes need to reflect the time symptoms began and what the signs and symptoms were, the actions taken, and the response of the client. Continuing assessments are also documented.
- Prepare for emergency cesarean birth.

Table 4–3 Characteristics of Placenta Previa and Abruptio Placentae

Placenta Previa	Abruptio Placentae
Bright red bleeding	May be bright red or dark red in color or no bleeding may be apparent if abruption is concealed.
No pain	May have no pain if abruption was on margin of placenta and has now resolved.
May have history of painless, bright red bleeding	May have pain if abruption is central (behind placenta). If contractions are present, may have increased tonus of uterus and poor uterine relaxation between contractions. Uterus may be "broadlike."

Evaluation

- The mother and baby are monitored carefully.
- Emergency measures are instituted immediately.

Abruptio Placentae in the Intrapartal Period

- Abruptio placentae is the premature separation of the placenta from the uterine wall.
- Signs and symptoms: see Table 4–3 for characteristics of placenta previa and abruptio placentae.
- Maternal risks:
    1. Maternal mortality rate is approximately 6%.
    2. Hemorrhage and development of DIC.
    3. Renal failure due to shock.
    4. Vascular spasm.
- Fetal/neonatal risks:
    1. Preterm labor.
    2. Anemia.
    3. Hypoxia.

Management of Abruptio Placentae

- Mild abruption (vaginal bleeding absent or external bleeding of less than 100 mL): the labor can continue and vaginal birth is anticipated.
- Moderate abruption (vaginal bleeding absent or from 100–500 mL) and severe abruption (vaginal bleeding absent or greater than 500 mL):
    1. Continuous monitoring of the mother and fetus.
    2. Monitoring and treatment of shock.
    3. Evaluation of coagulation.
    4. Possible blood replacement.
    5. Amniotomy and oxytocin infusion to augment labor or begin labor may be indicated.
- Cesarean birth is indicated when
    1. Fetal distress develops and a vaginal birth is not imminent.
    2. The fetus is alive and a severe abruption occurs.
    3. Hemorrhage becomes severe and threatens the life of the mother.
    4. Labor is not progressing.

Nursing Assessments for Abruptio Placentae

- Assess maternal history for associated factors:
    1. Pregnancy-induced hypertension (PIH).
    2. High multiparity.
    3. Trauma.
    4. Use of illicit drugs such as cocaine or crack.
- Assess type and amount of bleeding to assist in differentiating among possible causes of bleeding.
- Pads may be weighed to assess blood loss more accurately (1 g equals 1 mL). Hemorrhage of 500 mL or more increases chance of fetal death.
- Assess whether pain is present:
    1. Pain is present in most women with abruptio placentae.

    2. The pain is usually of sudden onset, is constant, and is localized to the uterus or the lower back.

    3. Determine if the pain is associated with uterine contractions. Is there pain between contractions (feels as if the uterus stays tight and does not relax)?

    4. Determine if there are tender areas over the uterus.

- Assess uterine contractions for frequency, duration, intensity, and resting tone between contractions. (Abruptio placentae is associated with a rising uterine tone baseline.)
- Assess size of uterus. If bleeding is concealed, the uterus may be filling with blood and the fundus will rise.
- Assess labor progress for cervical dilatation, effacement, and fetal station. (Abruption may be associated with precipitous birth.)
- Assess maternal vital signs.
- Assess fetal status by EFM.
- Assess laboratory studies (hemoglobin, hematocrit, DIC screen).

Nursing Diagnoses

- Fluid volume deficit related to hypovolemia secondary to excessive blood loss.
- Anxiety related to concern for personal health and the baby's safety.

Nursing Interventions for Abruptio Placentae

- Monitor maternal status. *Be alert for* beginning signs of shock (decreased BP, increased pulse, increased respirations).
- Monitor fetal status. *Be alert for* FHR baseline changes and late decelerations with decreased variability.
- Monitor amount of blood loss:
  1. Measure blood loss.
  2. Wear disposable gloves when handling blood-soaked items or while cleansing blood from woman.

- Carefully monitor labor status. *Be alert for* increased uterine tonus, which may be exhibited by
  1. Increased frequency of contractions (<2 minutes).
  2. Increased intensity.
  3. Incomplete uterine relaxation between contractions.
  4. Tenderness of the uterine fundus.
  5. A rising baseline of EFM strip.
- Monitor urine output. Urine output is reflective of circulatory status.
  1. Urine output needs to be at least 30 mL/hour.
  2. An indwelling bladder catheter will assist in monitoring urine output accurately.
  3. Amount of output is measured every 1 to 4 hours, depending on the severity of the bleeding.
- Monitor size of abdomen:
  1. Place measuring tape under woman; then bring it around to the front and over the umbilicus.
  2. Use either the upper or lower edge of the umbilicus and, for consistency, consider making marks on the maternal abdomen with a felt-tip pen to ensure consistent placement of the tape in each measurement.
- Monitor oxytocin if it is being administered. See discussion of induction of labor later in this chapter.
- Monitor laboratory studies. *Be alert for* development of consumption coagulopathy (DIC) as evidenced by decreasing platelets and fibrinogen and increased fibrin split products (see Table 4–4).
- Monitor oxygen status by pulse oximetry (pulse oximetry needs to be 95 or above). If reading is below 95, administer oxygen by face mask at 7–10 L/min.
- Monitor fluid and blood replacement.
- Monitor for signs of decreased platelet count such as purpura, petechiae, bruising, hematemesis, and rectal bleeding.
- Prepare for cesarean birth if vaginal birth is not imminent.
- Follow body substance isolation and Centers for Disease Control and Prevention (CDC) precautions at all times of exposure to body fluids.

Table 4–4   Laboratory Findings Associated with DIC

Lab Test	Normal Value	Value in DIC
Partial thromboplastin	60–70 sec	Prolonged
Platelets	150,000–400,000 μL	Decreased
Fibrinogen	200–400 mg/dL	Decreased
Fibrin degradation products (also called fibrin split products or fibrin)	2–10 μg/mL	Increased

- Provide emotional support for woman and her support team.
- Review the following critical aspects of the care you have provided:
  1. Are the woman's vital signs stable?
  2. Are the vital signs responding in an anticipated way to the medical therapy?
  3. What does the woman say about her condition?
  4. Is she anxious?
  5. Is the amount of bleeding increasing?
  6. What are the measured amounts of blood loss?
  7. Is there bleeding from any other site?
  8. Is the uterus becoming more tender, more sensitive?
  9. Is there a rising uterine resting tone?
  10. Is there a better position to place the woman in to maximize circulation and comfort?
  11. What other information do the woman and her loved ones need?
  12. Has there been a change in her consciousness level?

Sample Nurse's Charting

Uterine contractions every 3 min, 60 sec duration and strong intensity. Uterus relaxes between contractions. Client reports slight tenderness in the upper uterine fundus on the right when palpated. FHR 140–146, decreased variability, no accelerations with fetal movement. Deceleration of 15 bpm lasting 15 sec begins just after acme of each contraction. O_2 per face mask at 8 L/min. Client lying on left side. BP stable at 112/70. Admitting BP 114/72. Pulse 80 and regular. 100 cc dark red vaginal bleeding present on chux in last hour. Client breathing with contractions and relaxing well with encouragement. Partner provides continuous, ongoing support. Dr. Jones here with client. P. Gomez, RNC

Evaluation

- The woman and her baby have a safe labor and birth without further complications.
- The woman and family verbalize understanding of reasons for medical therapy and risks.

Placenta Previa in the Intrapartal Period

- In placenta previa the placenta is implanted in the lower uterine segment rather than the upper portion of the uterus.
- Placenta previa may occur as
  1. Low placental implantation.
  2. Partial or marginal previa.
  3. Complete previa.
- Maternal risks:
  1. Hemorrhage.
  2. Possible complications of emergency cesarean birth.
- Fetal/neonatal risks:
  1. Anemia due to maternal blood loss.
  2. Hypoxia due to maternal blood loss.

Management of Placenta Previa

- Diagnosis made from ultrasound examination.
- Cesarean birth scheduled if complete previa, gestation >37 weeks, and documented fetal maturity.
- Labor and vaginal birth may be possible if marginal placenta previa.

Nursing Assessments for Placenta Previa

- Assess type and amount of bleeding (see Table 4–3 for characteristics of placenta previa and abruptio placentae).
- Assess maternal vital signs and fetal status.
- Assess labor progress (uterine contraction frequency, duration, and intensity; fetal descent).
- Assess laboratory findings.

Nursing Diagnoses

- Risk for altered tissue perfusion related to blood loss.
- Risk for impaired fetal gas exchange related to decreased blood volume and hypotension.
- Anxiety related to concern for own personal status and the baby's safety.

Nursing Interventions for Placenta Previa

- Monitor bleeding. Weigh all absorbent pads to determine amount of blood loss.
- Monitor maternal vital signs for signs of shock.
- Monitor FHR for evidence of normality (baseline stable, variability average, no periodic decelerations or early decelerations).
- *Note* signs of possible fetal problems such as rising or falling baseline, decreased variability, and late and/or variable decelerations.
- Monitor laboratory studies.
   1. *Be alert for* evidence of decreasing hemoglobin and hematocrit.
   2. Coagulation problems are not as common with placenta previa as with abruptio placentae.
- Administer and monitor IV fluids and blood replacement.
- Monitor oxygen status. If vital signs are unstable or questionable, monitor pulse oximetry. If pulse oximetry is below 95, administer oxygen by face mask at 7–10 L/min.
- Maintain on bed rest with bathroom privileges.

- Provide emotional support to mother and support team.

Evaluation

- Maternal hemorrhage ceases and any hypovolemia is corrected as indicated by normal blood studies and normal maternal vital signs.
- Signs of fetal distress are recognized promptly, and corrective measures are begun.

Diabetes Mellitus in the Intrapartum Period

- Diabetes mellitus (DM) is an endocrine disorder of carbohydrate metabolism resulting from inadequate production or use of insulin. It may be a preexisting condition or may develop during pregnancy (gestational diabetes mellitus [see Chapter 2]).
- Maternal risks:
    1. Increased incidence of PIH.
    2. Hypoglycemia.
    3. Infection.
    4. Diabetic ketoacidosis.
    5. Hypertension.
    6. Prolonged labor due to cephalopelvic disproportion.
    7. Prolapsed cord related to hydramnios.
    8. Hypertonic contractions.
    9. Amniotic fluid embolism.
    10. Postpartum hemorrhage due to uterine atony.
- Fetal/neonatal risks:
    1. Fetal macrosomia.
    2. Birth trauma related to fetal macrosomia.
    3. Increase of congenital abnormalities.
    4. Fetal distress related to decreased uteroplacental function.
    5. Intrauterine fetal demise.

Intrapartal Management of Diabetes Mellitus

- Induction of labor at 40 weeks if labor does not begin spontaneously.
- Intravenous therapy with 5% dextrose in lactated Ringer's solution.
- Insulin infusion (rate determined by plasma glucose levels).
- Blood glucose levels every hour.
- Continuous electronic fetal monitoring.
- Assessment for CPD.
- Neonatologist present at birth.

Intrapartal Nursing Assessments for Diabetes Mellitus

- Review woman's prenatal record for the following:
  1. Fetal gestational age.
  2. Lecithin-sphingomyelin (L/S) ratio and presence of prostaglandin (PG).
  3. Degree of glycemic control.
  4. Medical or obstetrical complications.
- Monitor blood glucose levels hourly or as ordered.
- Assess FHR continuously with EFM.
- Assess labor progress—uterine contractions, cervical changes, and fetal descent.
- Assess for signs of PIH.
- Following childbirth, assess for uterine atony.

Nursing Diagnoses

- Fear related to impact of diabetes on maternal and fetal well-being.
- Risk for complications related to hypoglycemia or hyperglycemia.
- Altered uteroplacental tissue perfusion related to diabetic vascular changes.

Intrapartal Nursing Interventions for Diabetes Mellitus

- Monitor blood glucose via finger sticks.
- Observe for signs of hypoglycemia or hyperglycemia.
- Regulate IV per physician's orders.
- Regulate insulin therapy per physician's orders.
- Maintain woman in side-lying position to increase uteroplacental flow.
- Evaluate labor progress for failure to progress or evidence of CPD.
- Evaluate EFM tracing for late deceleration and/or decreased variability.
- Assess newborn for congenital problems.
- Reassure woman and her support team.

Evaluation

- Woman experiences decreased anxiety related to her health and her baby's health status.
- Woman's blood glucose levels remain within normal ranges.
- FHR is within normal limits, with average variability and no late decelerations.

Preeclampsia-Eclampsia in the Intrapartum Period

- Preeclampsia-eclampsia (sometimes called pregnancy-induced hypertension [PIH]) is a hypertensive disorder of pregnancy.
- Signs and symptoms:
  1. Hypertension.
  2. Proteinuria.
  3. Edema.
  4. Hyperreflexia.
  5. Headaches.

6. Visual disturbances.
7. Seizures.
- Maternal risks:
  1. Cerebral hemorrhage, edema, and thrombosis.
  2. Thrombocytopenia.
  3. Pulmonary edema.
  4. Oliguria and renal failure.
  5. Hepatic injury.
  6. Seizures and coma.
  7. Abruptio placentae.
  8. Disseminated intravascular coagulation (DIC).
- Fetal/neonatal risks:
  1. Intrauterine growth restriction (IUGR).
  2. Fetal distress related to placental insufficiency or abruptio placentae.
  3. Preterm birth.

Intrapartal Management of Preeclampsia-Eclampsia

1. Begin intravenous magnesium therapy.
2. Evaluate fetal status.
3. Monitor blood pressure and reflexes.
4. Ensure pediatrician or neonatal practitioner is present at birth.

Intrapartal Nursing Assessments for Preeclampsia-Eclampsia

- Assess uterine contraction pattern.
- Assess FHR.
- Assess vital signs.
- Assess deep tendon reflexes (DTRs).
- Assess level of consciousness.
- Assess intake and output.
- Assess degree of edema.

- Assess urinary protein with each voiding.

Nursing Diagnoses

- Risk for injury related to the possibility of seizures secondary to cerebral vasospasm or edema.
- Injury to fetus related to uteroplacental insufficiency.
- Fluid volume excess related to renal injury.

Intrapartal Nursing Interventions for Preeclampsia-Eclampsia

- Start and monitor IV magnesium sulfate therapy by infusion pump. (See Drug Guide: Magnesium Sulfate, page 273.)
- Piggyback magnesium sulfate line into main line.
- Observe for signs of magnesium toxicity (decreased respirations, diminished or absent reflexes, drooling, difficulty swallowing, marked lethargy).
- Have calcium gluconate at bedside as antidote for magnesium sulfate overdose.
- Maintain intake and output record.
- Chart blood pressure, respirations, and reflexes every hour.
- Obtain magnesium blood levels per physician's orders.
- Maintain a quiet, dark labor room.

Evaluation

- The woman suffers no eclamptic seizures.
- The woman gives birth to a healthy newborn.

Induction of Labor

- Induction is the stimulation of uterine contractions before the spontaneous onset of labor.
- Indications for induction:
    1. Diabetes mellitus.
    2. Renal disease.

   3. Preeclampsia-eclampsia.

   4. Premature rupture of membranes.

   5. History of precipitous labor and birth.

   6. Chorioamnionitis.

   7. Postterm gestation.

   8. Mild abruptio placentae with no fetal distress.

   9. Intrauterine fetal demise (IUFD).

  10. IUGR.

  11. Rh isoimmunization.

- Contraindications for induction:

   1. Client refusal.

   2. Placenta previa or vasa previa.

   3. Transverse fetal lie.

   4. Prior classic uterine incision.

   5. Active genital herpes infection.

   6. Some instances of positive human immunodeficiency virus (HIV) status.

   7. CPD.

   8. Severe fetal stress or distress; presence of FHR late decelerations.

- Maternal risks:

   1. Water intoxication.

   2. Rapid labor and birth.

   3. Cervical, vaginal, and/or perineal lacerations.

- Fetal/neonatal risks:

   1. Rapid intracranial pressure changes if rapid labor and birth occur.

   2. Decreased placental-fetal circulation if labor pattern is overstimulated.

- The most frequent methods of induction are amniotomy, intravenous administration of oxytocin, or both.

- Prostaglandin E_2 is currently being used for labor priming (softening of the cervix) at term but is not used to induce labor at that time. (See Drug

Guide: Dinoprostone (Cervidil) Vaginal Insert, page 270.)

- For oxytocin induction 1000 mL of solution (such as lactated Ringer's) is started IV by a large-bore plastic IV catheter (18 or 20 gauge). Ten units of Pitocin are added to a second 1000-mL bottle of IV fluid (second bottle needs to match the other primary IV). The IV containing the Pitocin is the secondary bottle, and this bottle is administered via an infusion pump.

Nursing Assessments during Induction of Labor

- Assess woman's knowledge and understanding regarding the induction procedure, associated nursing care, and the risks and benefits.
- Assess for any contraindications to the induction procedure.
- Assess maternal vital signs to provide a baseline for further assessments.
- Assess FHR characteristics after obtaining a 20-minute EFM strip.
- Assess FHR for reassuring characteristics (baseline 120–160 bpm, average variability, accelerations with fetal movement, no late or variable decelerations present).
- Assess maternal vital signs, contraction pattern and characteristics, cervical dilatation, and fetal response to IV oxytocin once infusion has begun and with each planned increase in the infusion rate.
- Assess maternal physiologic and psychologic response to uterine contractions.

Nursing Diagnoses

- Health-seeking behavior: information about induction related to an expressed desire to understand the procedure and its implications.

- Risk for altered placental tissue perfusion related to potential hypertonic contraction pattern.

Nursing Interventions during Induction of Labor

- Provide information to meet knowledge needs of woman and her partner.
- Prepare IV solution and obtain equipment for induction.
- Administer oxytocin as a secondary infusion and increase infusion pump rate according to CNM or physician order.
- Monitor contraction and cervical dilatation pattern and EFM tracing.
   1. If contractions occur more frequently than every 2 minutes, decrease the infusion rate.
   2. If fetal stress occurs (decreasing variability, decreasing baseline, or presence of late decelerations), discontinue oxytocin infusion and infuse primary IV solution, institute supportive nursing care (assist to side-lying position, monitor for hypotension, and initiate oxygen), and notify CNM or physician of adverse effects.
- Monitor maternal vital signs, contraction pattern, cervical dilatation status, and EFM tracing on a periodic basis and prior to any increase of oxytocin.
- Provide supportive nursing measures to increase maternal comfort.
- Advocate for the laboring woman when she requests analgesia or anesthesia block.
- Advise CNM or physician of maternal and fetal conditions frequently.
- Carefully evaluate the need for changes in the infusion rate of oxytocin (increase, decrease, or maintain rate) once an active labor pattern is present.

Evaluation

- Woman verbalizes understanding of the medication utilized, the need to take vital signs frequently, and the need for continuing fetal monitoring to evaluate contractions and fetal response.

- Woman experiences contraction pattern that remains within normal limits.

Obstetric Procedure: External Version

- Version is done to change the fetal presentation from breech to cephalic. It is usually scheduled in the 38th week of pregnancy but may be done in the 39th or 40th.

Nursing Assessments during External Version

- Assess the mother for presence of contraindications (nonreactive nonstress test [NST], evidence of CPD, multiple gestation, oligohydramnios, ruptured amniotic membranes, and placenta previa).
- Assess maternal BP, pulse, and respirations
- Assess fetal heart rate (establish presence of reassuring characteristics: FHR baseline between 120–160 bpm, moderate to average variability, absence of late or variable decelerations).

Nursing Diagnosis

- Health-seeking behavior: information about external version related to an expressed desire to understand the procedure, its risks, and its benefits.

Nursing Interventions during External Version

- Provide information regarding the version.
- Determine woman's Rh status. If she is Rh negative, obstetrician will probably order a minidose of Rh immune globulin (RhoGAM).
- Monitor maternal BP and pulse prior to the version and every 5 minutes during the procedure.
- Administer tocolytic per physician order.
- Monitor fetal heart rate continuously during the version.
- Provide support to the woman and her partner.

- Provide aftercare instructions that may include maternal monitoring for contractions and fetal movement (fetal kick counts).

Evaluation

- The version is accomplished successfully, with no complications.

Obstetric Procedure: Forceps-Assisted Birth

- Indications:
  1. Used for rotation of the fetus when there is a persistent posterior position or transverse arrest (anterior-posterior diameters of the fetal head remain transverse in the maternal pelvis).
  2. Used for traction to assist birth.
- Contraindications:
  1. CPD.
  2. Incomplete dilatation of the cervix.
  3. Unengaged fetal head.
- Maternal risks:
  1. Laceration of the cervix, vagina, or perineum.
  2. Hematoma.
  3. Extension of episiotomy into rectum.
  4. Rupture of uterus.
- Fetal/neonatal risks:
  1. Facial edema and/or bruising.
  2. Neurologic injury related to skull fracture or intracranial hemorrhage.

Nursing Assessments during Forceps-Assisted Birth

- Assess maternal ability to relax perineal muscles during forceps application and use.
- Assess maternal vital signs.

- Assess contraction pattern.
- Assess fetal status.
- Assess for contraindications.

Nursing Diagnoses

- Knowledge deficit related to lack of understanding of the procedure and its possible complications.
- Ineffective individual coping related to unexpected labor progress and use of procedure.

Nursing Interventions during Forceps-Assisted Birth

- Explain procedure to mother and partner.
- Monitor woman's comfort and coping level.
- Monitor uterine contractions and inform physician of presence of contractions.
- Monitor FHR after each contraction or continuously by EFM.
- Provide emotional support for the woman and her partner.
- Assess newborn immediately after birth for possible injuries related to forceps-assisted birth.

Evaluation

- Mother and partner understand procedure and possible complications.
- Mother and baby experience no complications.

Obstetric Procedure: Vacuum-Assisted Birth (Vacuum Extraction)

- Vacuum-assisted birth is an obstetric procedure used to facilitate the birth of a fetus.
- Indications: used for traction to assist birth.
- Contraindications:
  1. CPD.
  2. Face or breech presentation.

- Fetal/neonatal risks:
  1. Fetal scalp bruising and/or blistering.
  2. Cerebral trauma.
- Procedure:
  1. The physician places a suction cup on the fetal scalp.
  2. Tubing from the suction cup is attached to the suction device.
  3. The nurse usually initiates suction.
  4. The physician applies traction during contractions.
  5. Suction pressure is decreased between contractions.
- Nursing assessments, diagnoses, interventions, and evaluation are similar to those in forceps-assisted birth.

References

Cunningham, F. G., MacDonald, P. C., Gant, N. F., Leveno, K. J., Gilstrap, L. C., Hankins, G. C. V., and Clark, L. L. (1997). *Williams obstetrics* (20th ed.). Stamford, CT: Appleton & Lange.

Chapter 5

The Normal Newborn

At the moment of birth, numerous physiologic adaptations begin to take place in the newborn's body. Because of these dramatic changes, the newborn requires close observation to determine how smoothly she or he is making the transition to extrauterine life. The newborn also requires care that enhances her or his chances of making the transition successfully.

The broad goals of nursing care during this period are to provide comprehensive care to the newborn while she or he is in the nursery, to teach parents how to care for their new baby, and to support parenting efforts so that parents feel confident and competent.

Transitional Period

The transitional period involves three periods, called the first period of reactivity, sleep phase, and second period of reactivity. The characteristics of each period demonstrate the newborn's progression to independent functioning.

First Period of Reactivity

The first period of reactivity lasts for approximately 30 minutes after birth.

Characteristics

1. The newborn's vital signs are as follows: rapid apical pulse rate and irregular in rhythm. Respiratory rate as high as 80 breaths/minute, irregular, and some may be labored, with nasal flaring, expiratory grunting, and retractions.
2. Color fluctuates from pale pink to cyanotic.

3. Bowel sounds are usually absent, and the baby usually does not void or have a bowel movement during this period.

4. The newborn has minimal amounts of mucus at this time, a rigorous cry, and strong suck reflex. *Special tip:* During this period, the newborn's eyes are open more than they will be again for days. It is an excellent time for the attachment process to begin because the newborn is able to maintain eye contact for long periods of time.

Care Needs Specific to First Period of Reactivity

1. Assess and monitor heart rate and respirations q30 min for the first 4 hours after birth.

2. Keep baby warm (axillary or skin probe temperature between 36.5°C and 37°C [97.7°F–98.6°F]) with warmed blankets or overhead warming lights.

3. Place mother and baby together skin to skin to facilitate attachment.

4. Delay instillation of eye prophylactic for first hour to promote newborn-parent interaction.

Sleep Phase

The sleep phase begins about 30 minutes after the first period of reactivity and may last from a minute to 2 to 4 hours.

Characteristics

1. As the baby moves into the sleep phase, the heart rate and respirations decrease. While asleep, the respiratory rate and the apical pulse rate return to baseline values.

2. Skin color stabilizes; some acrocyanosis may be present. Bowel sounds become audible.

Care needs specific to sleep phase: The baby does not respond to external stimuli, but the mother and father can still enjoy holding and cuddling their baby.

Second Period of Reactivity

The second period of reactivity lasts about 4 to 6 hours.

Characteristics

1. Baby has intense sensitivity to internal and environmental stimuli. Apical pulse ranges from 120 to 160 bpm and can vary from bradycardia (<120 bpm) to tachycardia (>160 bpm). Respiratory rate (RR) is 30 to 60 breaths/minute with periods of more rapid respirations, but respirations remain unlabored (no nasal flaring or retractions).

2. Skin color fluctuates from pink or ruddy to mildly cyanotic with periods of mottling.

3. Baby often voids and passes meconium during this period.

4. Mucous secretions increase and the baby may gag on secretions. Sucking reflex is again strong, and baby may be very active.

Care Needs Specific to Second Period of Reactivity

1. Close observation of newborn for possible choking on the excessive mucus normally present. Use bulb syringe to remove mucus and teach parents how to use the bulb syringe.

2. Observe for any episode of apnea and initiate methods of stimulation if needed (eg, stroke baby's back, turn baby to side).

3. Assess baby's interest in (sucking, rooting, and swallowing) and ability to feed (no choking or gagging during feeding, no vomiting of feeding in unchanged form).

Additional Assessments and Interventions in the Transitional Period

In these first few hours of life, the nurse will accomplish the following:

1. Monitor newborn vital signs. See Table 5–1 for summary of normal findings. (See Appendix F for additional information regarding selected newborn laboratory values.)

2. Weigh the newborn and measure length, head, and chest circumference (see Table 5–2 and Figure 5–1). To

Table 5–1 Key Signs of Newborn Transition

Pulse: 120–160 beats/min
During sleep as low as 100 beats/min; if crying, up to 180 beats/min
Respirations: 30–60 respirations/min
Predominantly diaphragmatic but synchronous with abdominal movements
Brief periods of apnea (5–10 sec), with no color or heart rate changes
Temperature
    Axillary: 36.5°C–37°C (97.5°F–98.6°F)
    Skin: 36°C–36.5°C (96.8°F–97.5°F)
Blood glucose: above 40 mg/dL
Hematocrit: less than 65%–70% central venous sample
Blood pressure: 80–60/45–40 mm Hg at birth; 100/50 mm Hg at day 10

Table 5–2 Newborn Weight and Measurements

Weight
Average: 3405 g (7 lb, 8 oz)
Range: 2500–4000 g (5 lb, 8 oz, to 8 lb, 13 oz)
Weight is influenced by racial origin and maternal age and size
Length
Average: 50 cm (20 in)
Range: 48–52 cm (18–22 in)
Growth: 2.0 cm (1 in) per month for first 6 months
Head Circumference
Average: 32–37 cm (12½–14½ in)
Approximately 2 cm (about 1 in) larger than chest circumference

determine length, place the newborn flat on the back with legs extended as much as possible. Hold the head still at the top of the measuring tape and gently stretch the legs downward toward the bottom of the tape (see Figure 5–2). To measure head circumference place the tape over the most prominent part of the occiput and bring it around above the eyebrows (see Figure 5–3). The circumference of the head is approximately 2 cm greater than the circumference of the chest at birth.

Figure 5–1
Weighing of newborns. The scale is balanced with the protective pad in place. The caregiver's hand is poised above the infant as a safety measure.

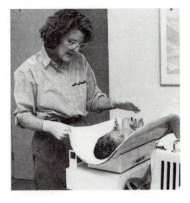

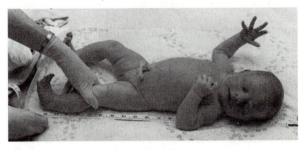

Figure 5–2   Measuring the length of the newborn.

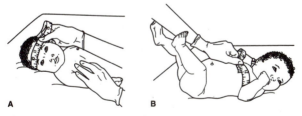

A   **B**

Figure 5–3   Obtaining newborn measurements.
A, Measuring the head circumference of the newborn. The tape is placed on the occiput and then brought around and placed just above the eyebrows. **B,** Measuring the chest circumference of the newborn. The tape is placed over the lower edge of the scapula and brought around to the front and placed over the nipple line.

To obtain chest circumference, place the tape measure at the lower edge of the scapulas and bring it around anteriorly over the nipple line.

3. Complete the gestational age assessment of the newborn during the first 4 hours of the newborn's life so that age-related problems can be identified. Clinical gestational age assessment tools have two components: external physical characteristics and neuromuscular status.

Physical characteristics (with the exception of sole creases) can be assessed over the first 24 hours. Neuromuscular development may be influenced by the newborn's unstable nervous system or labor and birth events. It can be assessed in the first 24 hours; however, if the findings drastically differ from the gestational age determined by looking at physical characteristics, the assessment may be repeated after 24 hours.

Method of Assessment

Use Newborn Maturity Rating and Classification (Figure 5–4). Assess each of the factors listed and assign a score of 0 to 5 for each one. It is helpful to circle the results for each assessment.

Physical Characteristics

- **Skin** in the preterm neonate appears thin and transparent, with veins prominent over the abdomen early in gestation. As term approaches, the skin appears opaque because of increased subcutaneous tissue. Disappearance of the protective vernix caseosa promotes skin desquamation (peeling).
- **Lanugo,** a fine hair covering, decreases as gestational age increases. The amount of lanugo is greatest at 28 to 30 weeks and then disappears, first from the face and then from the trunk and extremities.

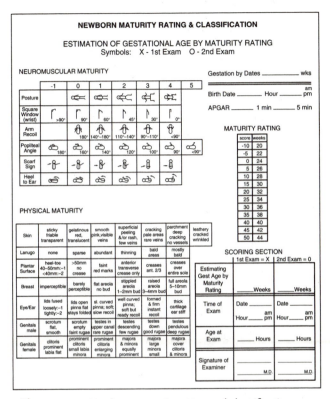

NEWBORN MATURITY RATING & CLASSIFICATION

ESTIMATION OF GESTATIONAL AGE BY MATURITY RATING
Symbols: X - 1st Exam   O - 2nd Exam

NEUROMUSCULAR MATURITY

	-1	0	1	2	3	4	5
Posture							
Square Window (wrist)	>90°	90°	60°	45°	30°	0°	
Arm Recoil		180°	140°–180°	110°–140°	90°–110°	<90°	
Popliteal Angle	180°	160°	140°	120°	100°	90°	<90°
Scarf Sign							
Heel to Ear							

Gestation by Dates _____ wks

Birth Date _____ Hour _____ am/pm

APGAR _____ 1 min _____ 5 min

MATURITY RATING

score	weeks
-10	20
-5	22
0	24
5	26
10	28
15	30
20	32
25	34
30	36
35	38
40	40
45	42
50	44

PHYSICAL MATURITY

Skin	sticky friable transparent	gelatinous red, translucent	smooth pink, visible veins	superficial peeling &/or rash, few veins	cracking pale areas rare veins	parchment deep cracking no vessels	leathery cracked wrinkled
Lanugo	none	sparse	abundant	thinning	bald areas	mostly bald	
Plantar Surface	heel-toe 40–50mm:–1 <40mm:–2	>50mm no crease	faint red marks	anterior transverse crease only	creases ant. 2/3	creases over entire sole	
Breast	imperceptible	barely perceptible	flat areola no bud	stippled areola 1–2mm bud	raised areola 3–4mm bud	full areola 5–10mm bud	
Eye/Ear	lids fused loosely:–1 tightly:–2	lids open pinna flat stays folded	sl. curved pinna; soft; slow recoil	well curved pinna; soft but ready recoil	formed & firm instant recoil	thick cartilage ear stiff	
Genitals male	scrotum flat, smooth	scrotum empty faint rugae	testes in upper canal rare rugae	testes descending few rugae	testes down good rugae	testes pendulous deep rugae	
Genitals female	clitoris prominent labia flat	prominent clitoris small labia minora	prominent clitoris enlarging minora	majora & minora equally prominent	majora large minora small	majora cover clitoris & minora	

SCORING SECTION

	1st Exam = X	2nd Exam = O
Estimating Gest Age by Maturity Rating	_____ Weeks	_____ Weeks
Time of Exam	Date _____ Hour _____ am/pm	Date _____ Hour _____ am/pm
Age at Exam	_____ Hours	_____ Hours
Signature of Examiner	_____ M.D.	_____ M.D.

Figure 5–4   Newborn maturity rating and classification. Source: Ballard, J. L., Khoury, J. C., Wedig, K., Wang, L., Eilers-Walsmann, B. L., & Lipp, R. (1991). New Ballard score, expanded to include extremely premature infants. *Journal Pediatrics, 119,* 417.

- **Sole (plantar creases)** needs to be assessed within 12 hours of birth because afterward the skin of the foot begins drying and superficial creases disappear. Development of sole creases begins at the top of the sole and proceeds downward toward the heel.

- **Areola** is inspected and the breast bud tissue is gently palpated to determine the size. It is important to place your index and middle finger over this tissue and roll over the breast bud to estimate the size, rather than pinching the tissue. Another method of measuring involves placing a ruler just above the breast bud tissue for more accurate measurement. Most experienced nurses have completed the assessment often enough that they can estimate the size very accurately.

- **Ear form and cartilage** change throughout gestation. By 36 weeks some cartilage and slight incurving of the upper pinna are present, and the pinna springs back slowly when folded.

  To assess, observe ear form and then fold the pinna of the ear forward against the side of the head, release it, and observe the results.

- **Genitals** change in appearance during gestation because of the amount of subcutaneous fat present. **Female genitals** at 30 to 32 weeks have a prominent clitoris, and the labia majora are small and widely separated. At 36 to 40 weeks the labia nearly cover the clitoris, and at more than 40 weeks the labia majora completely cover the clitoris. Complete the assessment by observation. **Male genitals** are evaluated for size of the scrotal sac, presence of rugae, and descent of the testes. Observe the size of the scrotal sac and the presence or absence of rugae. The scrotal sac can be gently palpated to determine descent of the testes.

Neuromuscular Characteristics

- **Resting posture** should be assessed as the baby lies undisturbed on a flat surface such as his or her bed.

- **Square window (wrist)** is elicited by flexing the baby's hand toward the ventral forearm. The angle formed at the wrist is measured (by estimation and matching it against the angles on the scoring tool) (see Figure 5–5).

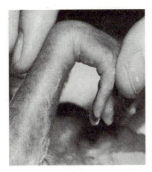

A

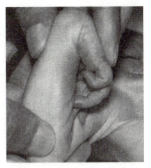

B

Figure 5–5 Square window sign. **A,** This angle is 90 degrees and suggests an immature newborn of 28 to 32 weeks' gestation. **B,** A 30-degree angle is commonly found from 39 to 40 weeks' gestation. **C,** A 0-degree angle can occur from 40 to 42 weeks. Source: Dubowitz, L., & Dubowitz, V. (1977). *The gestation age of the newborn.* Menlo Park, CA:

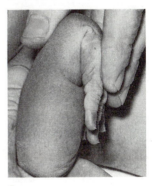

C

Addison-Wesley. Reprinted by permission of V. Dubowitz, MD, Hammersmith Hospital, London, England.

- **Arm recoil** is a test of flexion development. It is best evaluated after the first hour of life, when the baby has had time to recover from the stress of birth. To assess, place the newborn in a supine position (lying on the back), completely flex both elbows (by holding the newborn's hands and placing the hands up against the forearms), hold them in this position for about 5 seconds, and then release them. On release, the elbows of a full-term newborn form an angle of less than 90 degrees and rapidly recoil back to flexed position. The arms of a preterm newborn have slower recoil time and form greater than a 90-degree angle. Assessment of arm recoil should be bilateral to rule out brachial palsy.

- **Popliteal angle** is determined with the newborn flat on his or her back. Flex the thigh on the newborn's abdomen or chest and place the index finger of your other hand behind the newborn's ankle to extend the lower leg until resistance is met. Then measure the angle formed. Results vary from no resistance in the very immature infant to an 80-degree angle in the term infant.

- **Scarf sign** is elicited by placing the neonate supine and drawing an arm across the chest toward the infant's opposite shoulder until resistance is met. (Newborns need to remain lying on their backs. The location of the elbow is then noted in relation to the midline of the chest) (see Figure 5–6).

- **Heel to ear** is performed by placing the baby in a supine position and, while stabilizing the hip on the bed, gently drawing the foot toward the ear on the same side until resistance is felt. Both the degree of knee extension and the proximity of the foot to the ear are assessed. In a very preterm newborn, the leg will remain straight and the foot will go to the ear or beyond. With advancing gestational age the newborn demonstrates increasing resistance to this maneuver. If the newborn was in a breech presentation, this assessment should be delayed until the legs are positioned more normally.

Scoring

All individual scores are added and the total number is compared to the score on the Newborn Maturity Rating and Classification tool. A score of 35 equals 38 weeks, a score of 37 equals 39 weeks, and a score of 40 equals 40 weeks. The estimated gestational age is then plotted on a tool that classifies

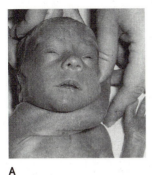

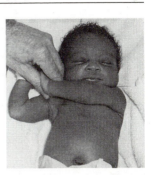

A   B

Figure 5–6   Scarf sign. **A,**
No resistance is noted until
after 30 weeks' gestation.
The elbow moves readily
past the midline. **B,** The
elbow is at midline at 36 to
40 weeks' gestation. **C,**
Beyond 40 weeks' gestation
the elbow will not reach the
midline. Source: Dubowitz,
L., & Dubowitz, V. (1977).
*The gestation age of the
newborn.* Menlo Park, CA:
Addison-Wesley. Reprinted by
permission of V. Dubowitz,
MD, Hammersmith Hospital,
London, England.

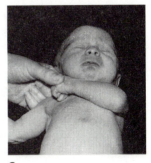

C

newborns by birth weight and gestational age (see Figure 5–7).
Most newborns are appropriate for gestational age (AGA). A
baby that is large for gestational age (LGA) or small for gestational age (SGA) may require additional assessment and intervention (for further discussion, see Chapter 6).

4. Administer erythromycin (Ilotycin) ointment (or silver
    nitrate drops) into the newborn's eyes. This is a legally
    required prophylactic eye treatment for *Neisseria*

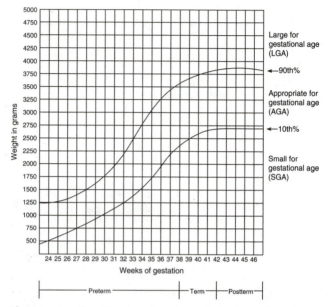

Figure 5–7 Classification of newborns by birth weight and gestational age. The nurse places the newborn's birth weight and gestational age on the graph and classifies the newborn as large for gestational age (LGA), appropriate for gestational age (AGA), or small for gestational age (SGA). Source: Battaglia, F. C., & Lubchenco, L. O. (1967). A practical classification of newborn infants by weight and gestational age. *Journal of Pediatrics, 71,* 161.

gonorrhoea, which may have infected the newborn during the birth process. Ilotycin has the advantage of being useful for treating both gonorrhea and chlamydia; it is also less irritating to the newborn's eyes, which results in decreased incidence of swelling and discharge. (See Drug Guide: Erythromycin Ophthalmic Ointment [Ilotycin Ophthalmic], on page 271.)

5. Administer prophylactic dose of vitamin K. Vitamin K is given to prevent hemorrhage, which can occur because of

Figure 5–8
Newborn injection sites. The middle third of the preferred site for intramuscular injection in the newborn.

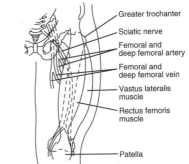

- Greater trochanter
- Sciatic nerve
- Femoral and deep femoral artery
- Femoral and deep femoral vein
- Vastus lateralis muscle
- Rectus femoris muscle
- Patella

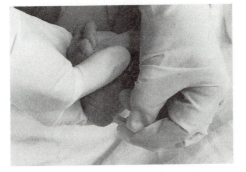

Figure 5–9 Blood is obtained by a heel stick for a glucose test.

low prothrombin levels in the first few days of life. (See Figure 5–8 for injection sites and Drug Guide: Vitamin K_1, Phytonadione [AquaMEPHYTON], on page 280.)

6. Assess glucose level. A drop of blood is obtained by heel stick and blood glucose is determined (see Figure 5–9). The glucose oxidase reagent strip or glucose oxidase analyzer should read >40 mg/dL; a value <40 mg/dL needs to be followed up by drawing a central blood sample (drawn from a vein in the hand or antecubital space) for further laboratory evaluation. Treatment is begun if

needed (see Chapter 6 for discussion of hypoglycemia). *Be alert for* hypoglycemia in high-risk babies such as SGA, infant of diabetic mother (IDM), AGA preterm, and any newborn who was stressed during labor and at birth. Outward signs of hypoglycemia may include lethargy, jitteriness, poor feeding, vomiting, pallor, apnea, irregular respirations, and/or tremors.

7. Maintain temperature through use of a controlled radiant warmer. A probe is placed on the newborn's abdomen just under the ribs or over the area of the liver. The probe indicates the newborn's temperature, and the radiant heater responds by becoming warmer or cooler. *Be alert for* newborns at risk for hypothermia (temperature <97.7°F), including preterms, SGA, and any baby who was stressed at birth. If the newborn's temperature is 36.5°C (97.7°F) or below (axillary or skin probe temperature), rewarming is needed. Place the baby under a radiant warmer, undressing him or her so that the skin can be warmed. When the skin probe indicates that the desired temperature has been reached, recheck axillary temperature. The baby may be removed from the warmer; however, axillary temperature should be rechecked about every 30 minutes until the baby has maintained a normal temperature for 2 hours. Successful transition to extrauterine existence is documented by stabilization of vital signs and establishment of awake-sleep cycles and feeding, stooling, and voiding patterns.

Posttransitional Nursing Care

Overview

Once the newborn has passed through the transitional period, the baby is transferred to a normal newborn area. Normal newborn care usually includes assessment of vital signs (axillary temperature, apical pulse, and respirations) every 4 hours, a physical assessment every 8 hours, application of a drying agent to the umbilical stump every 8 hours, feeding every 3 to 4 hours, diapering as needed, and weighing once every 24 hours.

Physical Assessment

It is usually easier to proceed from head to toe; however, you need to assess axillary temperature, apical pulse, and respirations while the baby is quiet. Completing the assessment in the mother's room provides a wonderful opportunity for teaching, sharing, and role modeling for first-time mothers.

1. **Head.** Palpate and observe fontanelles. The anterior fontanelle is the largest and is diamond shaped. The posterior fontanelle is triangular in shape. The sagittal suture (located on the top of the head, from front to back) is smooth and without ridges.

   Common variations: Bulging of fontanelle (increased intracranial pressure), depressed fontanelle (dehydration), overriding of sagittal suture (molding), caput succedaneum (edema in tissues from trauma), cephalhematoma (bleeding into the periosteal space).

   Be alert for premature closing of both anterior and posterior sutures (craniosynostosis), which requires further assessment.

2. **Eyes.** Inspect eyes and lids. Eyes should be clear, without drainage, and no swelling of eyelids. Subconjunctival hemorrhage may be present.

   Common variations: Swelling of eyelid (birth trauma, reaction to eye prophylaxis).

   Be alert for purulent drainage, an indication for further assessment for infection and treatment.

3. **Ears.** Inspect outer ear. A full-term baby has incurving of the top two-thirds of the pinna. The top of the ear should be above an imaginary line drawn from the inner canthus to the outer canthus of the eye and extended around toward the ear. Rotation of the ear should be in the midline and not tipped forward or backward.

   Be alert for low-set ears, which may be associated with a variety of congenital problems.

4. **Nose.** Inspect. Nares should be clear and without mucus. (Remember, newborn is an obligatory nose breather, so a

stuffy nose has much greater implications for a newborn baby.)

Common variations: none.

Be alert for presence of nasal flaring. If present, assess respiratory rate, retractions and grunting, and skin color. A pulse-oximeter determination may provide further information (reading should be above 90%).

5. **Mouth.** Inspect inside of mouth and palpate hard palate. Hard and soft palate should be intact (may visualize while the baby is crying or may palpate with an unpowdered gloved finger). (An opening indicates cleft palate.) Inspect gums for supernumerary teeth (these teeth usually do not cause a problem but may loosen and fall out unexpectedly).

Common variations: Supernumerary teeth and Epstein's pearls.

Be alert for an opening in the palate (cleft palate), which needs to be evaluated quickly. Presence of white patches on the mucous membranes that appear as milk deposits but cannot be wiped away with a 4×4 gauze pad may indicate thrush (*Candida albicans*). Excessive mucus may be associated with esophageal atresia.

6. **Chest.** Inspect. Chest should be symmetric. Breasts may be flat or slightly enlarged because of the effects of maternal estrogen (this may last about 1 week). Count respiratory rate over 1 minute (uncover baby and look at movement of chest or abdomen).

Common variations: Supernumerary nipple(s).

Be alert for retractions (intercostal or sternal). If they are present, assess respiratory rate and determine baby's need for oxygen.

7. **Heart.** Auscultate. Apical pulse ranges from 120 to 160 bpm but may be as low as 100 bpm with sleep. Auscultate apical rate for 1 full minute when the newborn is asleep. Palpate brachial, radial, femoral, and pedal pulses. Compare brachial pulses bilaterally and with the femoral pulses.

Common variations: A transitory murmur may be heard for the first few hours of life.

Be alert for bradycardia (<100 bpm) or tachycardia (>160 bpm).

8. **Abdomen.** Inspect, auscultate, and palpate. Abdomen should be flat to slightly rounded (without distention), and bowel sounds should be heard in all quadrants. Umbilical stump should be drying and have no redness, discharge, or bleeding.

   Be alert for bleeding and/or purulent drainage from cord, which require further assessment and treatment.

9. **Genitals.** Inspect. Genitals should be clearly differentiated. Both testes should be palpable in scrotum.

   Common variations: Pseudomenstruation (small amount vaginal bleeding) in female infants due to maternal estrogen exposure; clear mucus from the vagina; vaginal skin tag.

   Be alert for urinary meatus on the underside of the penis (hypospadias).

10. **Back.** Inspect. Back should be smooth, with no tufts of hair present over the lower back.

    Common variations: Mongolian spot over lower back.

11. **Hips.** Inspect and perform Ortolani's maneuver to rule out congenital dislocation of hips (hip dislocatability). Legs should be of equal length and the skin folds on both right and left posterior thighs should be symmetric (see Figure 5–10). To do Ortolani's maneuver, place newborn on her or his back. Place the palm of your right hand on the newborn's left knee and extend your index and middle finger toward the hip. Your fingertips should be on the top of the greater trochanter. Place your left hand in the same manner. With hips and knees flexed at a 90-degree angle, lift thigh to bring femoral head toward the acetabulum and apply gentle abduction. Feel for a "clunk" under your fingertips. If a clunk is felt, notify baby's care provider. The baby will most likely be placed in a Pavlik harness or abduction splint to keep the hip abducted.

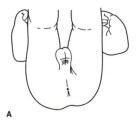

A

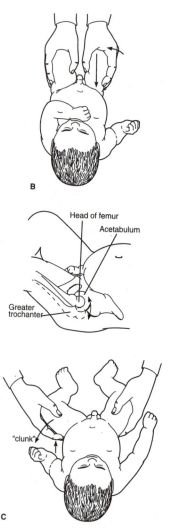

B

Head of femur

Acetabulum

Greater trochanter

"clunk"

C

Figure 5–10
A, Congenitally dislocated right hip in a young infant as seen on gross inspection.
B, Barlow's (dislocation) maneuver. Baby's thigh is grasped and adducted with gentle downward pressure. Dislocation is palpable as femoral head slips out of acetabulum.
C, Ortolani's maneuver puts downward pressure on the hip and then inward rotation. If the hip is dislocated, this forces the femoral head over the acetabular rim with a noticeable "clunk."
Source: Smith, D. W. (1981). *Recognizable patterns of human deformation.* Philadelphia: Saunders, 1981.

12. **Extremities.** Inspect. All extremities should be symmetric and move equally. Count digits on hands and feet; inspect palmar creases and for club foot. Note any webbing (syndactyly).

    Common variations: none.

    Be alert for asymmetric movement or no movement of an extremity, which needs to be reported and assessed further.

13. **Skin color.** Inspect. Ensure skin color is appropriate for ethnic grouping. Any evidence of acrocyanosis usually should have abated. Observe closely for signs of jaundice. Jaundice is first detectable on the face, the mucous membranes of the mouth, and the sclera. It is evaluated by blanching the tip of the nose, the forehead, the sterum, or the gum line. If jaundice is present, the area will appear yellowish immediately after blanching. Laboratory testing will verify the total bilirubin level.

    Common variations: Milia may be present over the nose. A variety of markings may be present on the skin (see Table 5–3).

    Be alert for cyanosis; it requires immediate reassessment and treatment. Pallor may be associated with anemia, and ruddiness may indicate an elevated hematocrit (>65%).

    Jaundice noted before 24 hours of age should be reported. Jaundice requires additional assessment, evaluation, and then treatment as needed. The jaundice may be treated with phototherapy.

14. **Elimination.** Note newborn record. Newborn should void and have a bowel movement within 24 hours after birth. After that, most babies have six to eight wet diapers a day and may stool at least once a day. Breastfed babies tend to have more frequent stools.

    Common variations: none.

    Be alert if baby does not void within 24 hours. Assess amount of fluid taken in and urethral opening. If no stool, assess abdomen for distention and bowel sounds. Diarrhea stools can be very serious for the newborn.

Table 5-3 Birthmarks

Type	Characteristics	Parent Teaching
Telangiectatic nevi (stork bites)	Pale pink or red flat dilated capillaries over eyelids, nose, and nape of neck	Seen more with crying Blanch easily, fade by 2 years of age, no clinical significance
Mongolian spots	Bluish-black macular areas over dorsal area and buttocks	Common in dark-skinned races Gradually fade in 1st to 2nd year of life Mistaken for bruises—must document in newborn chart
Nevus flammeus (port-wine stain)	Nonelevated, sharply outlined, red-purple dense area of capillaries, primarily on face In black infants may appear as a purple-black stain	Does not fade with time nor blanch as a rule Can cover with opaque cosmetic cream Suggestive of Sturge-Weber syndrome (involving 5th cranial nerve)

Observe stool characteristics closely and test the stool for occult blood (Hematest) and sugar loss (Clinitest or other glucose testing).

15. **Behavioral.** Observe. Baby quiets to soothing, cuddling, or wrapping. Moves through all sleep-awake states. When held in front of parent or caregiver, baby will turn head toward sound.

Common variations: none.

Be alert for excessive crying, fretfulness, and inability to quiet self, which may be associated with drug withdrawal in the neonate.

Tip: Completing the behavioral assessment in the mother's room provides a wonderful opportunity for learning about the individual baby's cues and personality.

Assessment of Reflexes

At some point during the time you spend with this newborn, assess normal newborn reflexes.

1. **Moro.** Elicited by startling the newborn with a loud noise or sudden movement. Newborn straightens arms and hands out while flexing knees. The arms then return to the chest as in an embrace. The fingers spread, forming a C, and the infant may cry.

2. **Grasp.** Elicited by stimulating the newborn's palm with a finger or object. The newborn grasps and holds the object or finger firmly enough to be lifted momentarily from the crib.

3. **Rooting.** Elicited when the side of the newborn's mouth or cheek is touched. In response, the newborn turns toward that side and opens the lips to suck.

Documentation of Assessment Findings and Care

Assessment findings may be recorded on computer charting systems, on neonatal flow sheets, or in narrative notes. A narrative note might be recorded as follows:

Anterior fontanelle soft and flat, posterior fontanelle palpated closed at this time, some molding present with overriding of sagittal suture, caput succedaneum over posterior aspect of head. Eyes clear and without discharge or swelling. Nares clear without flaring or discharge. Mouth clear, and palate intact. Chest movements symmetrical without retractions, apical pulse 134, regular, and no murmurs auscultated. Abdomen soft and nondistended. Bowel sounds × 4. Baby has had a meconium and transitional stool. Umbilical stump drying and without redness or discharge. No redness or discharge noted on genitalia. Perineal area cleansed and A and D ointment applied. Back clear. Moves all extremities equally. No hip click. Palmar creases normal. Skin color appropriate to ethnic group and without cyanosis. Soothes with cuddling and rocking. M. Chin, RNC

Additional Aspects of Newborn Daily Care

1. **Suctioning.** Achieved by compressing the bulb syringe, inserting it into the side of the mouth, and then releasing the bulb. The bulb should be withdrawn and the contents expelled onto a paper towel or cloth. The bulb is then recompressed and placed into the other side of the mouth if needed. It is best to have the bulb available at all times for the newborn. It is important to teach the parents the use of the bulb at their first contact with the baby. Some parents are frightened of the bulb, and it helps for them to actually hold it and compress it. When choking occurs, the baby may be picked up and held with the head slightly down and the mouth to the side to facilitate the drainage of mucus. It can be frightening to deal with a choking baby.

2. **Positioning.** Place the baby on the right side following feedings, with a rolled blanket at the back to hold the baby in this position. The baby can be placed on the back after the cord (and circumcision if done) heals and the baby is not regurgitating feedings.

3. **Swaddling.** The newborn seems to be comforted by being wrapped snugly in blankets (see Figure 5–11).

4. **Holding.** To pick up the newborn, take hold of the feet with one hand, and slide the other hand up under the baby until you reach the back of the shoulders and neck. The baby can now be picked up and placed up over your

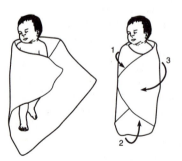

Figure 5–11 Steps used for swaddling a baby.

shoulder or cradled in the crook of your arm.
(Sometimes it is easier to place the baby against your
shoulder first, get settled, and then change the baby to
the crook of your arm. If you are right handed, you will
tend to be most comfortable cradling the baby in your
left arm. Remember to teach new parents this technique.) The baby may also be held in a football hold.

5. **Circumcision care.** Some parents choose to have their
male newborn circumcised. Prior to the procedure, the
parents need to validate that they understand the procedure and sign an informed consent form. Some form of
analgesia Emla cream, dorsal penile nerve block, or subcutaneous ring block is recommended. After the circumcision, the penis needs to be assessed for bleeding. If a
clamp or Plastibell is used, A and D ointment, petroleum
jelly, or antibiotic ointment is applied at each diaper
change to provide protection to the skin and keep the
penis from sticking to the diaper. If a Plastibell is used,
the remaining plastic ring protects the penis. Other than
cleansing by letting warm water softly rinse over the penis to clear away urine and patting it dry, no other care is
required. The Plastibell usually falls off by itself. If it is
still in place after 8 days, the parents need to contact
their care provider.

   Comfort measures immediately after the circumcision
may include wrapping the baby in soft blankets and rocking, walking with the baby, using a pacifier, feeding after
initial crying has abated, singing, gently rubbing the back,
talking to the baby, and using therapeutic touch (use
short, light, feathery strokes for a short period of time).

6. **Testing for phenylketonuria (PKU).** Prior to the newborn's discharge, blood needs to be obtained by heel stick
for PKU testing. The newborn needs to be at least 24
hours old for a valid test (Wallman, 1998). A second test
will be done in 7 to 14 days, and it is important to stress
the need for the second test with the parents. It is usually
done on an outpatient basis.

7. **Recombinant hepatitis B vaccine.** Universal hepatitis B
vaccination for all infants, regardless of maternal HBsAg

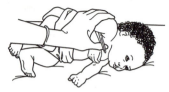

Figure 5–12 The axillary temperature should be taken for 3 minutes. The newborn's arm should be tightly but gently pressed against the thermometer and the newborn's side.

status, is currently recommended by the Centers for Disease Control and Prevention (CDC) and American Academy of Pediatrics (Selekman, 2000). Infants born to HBsAg-positive mothers should receive hepatitis B vaccine and HBIG within 12 hours of birth.

Parent Education

Provide information as needed on the following topics:

1. **Axillary temperature.** Place the thermometer in the baby's right or left axilla. The thermometer needs to be in contact with skin on all sides (see Figure 5–12). Hold the thermometer in place for 3 minutes unless an electronic thermometer is used. It is important to keep your hand on the thermometer at all times to ensure correct placement and prevent an accident. After reading the temperature, cleanse the thermometer by rinsing in cool water and wiping with a soft towel. Review normal range of temperature (axillary: 97.8° to 99°F). **Teaching tip:** Ask parents what type of thermometer they will be using and plan your teaching to that specific type. This may be done in the birthing center and reinforced in the home during a home visit (see Chapter 9).

2. **Diapering with reusable cloth diapers.** Many diaper-folding methods are available, as well as diaper wraps that allow the diaper to be placed inside a Velcro-fastened wrapper (see Figure 5–13). Handwashing prior to and after changing the diaper is essential.

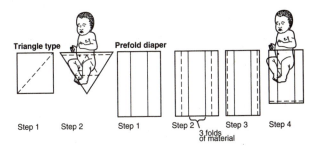

Figure 5–13   Two methods of using cloth diapers.

3. **Diapering with single-use paper diapers.** The baby is placed on the diaper, the front is pulled up toward the navel, and the sides are brought forward and attached by a sticky tab to the front of the diaper. Care needs to be followed to fold the diaper below the level of the umbilicus for the first 7 to 10 days. In addition, soiled diapers should not be left in open waste containers. Handwashing prior to and after changing the diaper is essential.

4. **When to call a health care provider.** The parents should call their health care provider if any of the following conditions occurs:
   - Water-loss stools (small amount of stool surrounded by a ring of water in the diaper).
   - Axillary temperature of >101°F or <97.6°F.
   - Any color change involving pallor or cyanosis.
   - Increasing jaundice (yellow tone) of the skin.
   - Pustules, rashes, or blisters other than normal newborn rash.
   - Refusal of two feedings in a row.
   - More than one episode of forceful vomiting or frequent vomiting (over 6 hours), especially projectile.
   - Abdominal distention, crying when trying to pass stools, or absence of stools after stool pattern is established.

- No wet diapers for 18 to 24 hours or fewer than six wet diapers per day after 4 days of age.
- Discharge or bleeding from umbilical cord, circumcision, or any opening (except vaginal mucus or pseudomenstruation).
- Inconsolable infant (quieting techniques are not effective) or continuous high-pitched cry.
- Lethargy (listlessness), difficulty in awakening baby.

References

Selekman, J. (2000). Immunization schedule 2000. *Pediatric Nursing, 26*(2), 209–210.

Wallman, C. M. (1998). Newborn genetic screening. *Neonatal Network, 17*(3), 55–60.

Chapter 6

The At-Risk Newborn

Hypoglycemia

Overview

Hypoglycemia is a condition of abnormally low levels of serum glucose. It can be defined as a blood glucose level below 40 mg/dL after birth for all newborns, or a glucose oxidase reagent strip reading below 45 mg/dL when corroborated by a blood glucose test. Newer techniques, such as using a glucose oxidase analyzer or an optical bedside glucose analyzer (eg, One Touch), are more reliable for bedside screening because interpreting the color is not as subjective. In clinical practice, an infant with a blood glucose level less than 40 mg/dL requires intervention. Also, plasma glucose values <20 to 25 mg/dL should be treated with parenteral glucose, regardless of the age or gestation.

Presentation of symptoms and blood glucose levels vary greatly with each baby. Symptoms usually occur at <40 mg/dL and appear between 24 and 72 hours after birth or within 6 hours after birth in severely stressed infants. A glucose level of 45 mg/dL or more by 72 hours of age is the goal regardless of weight, gestational age, or other predisposing factors. Clinical manifestations vary greatly but can include tremors or jittery movements, irritability, lethargy or hypotonia, irregular respirations, apnea, cyanosis, pallor, refusal to suck or poor feeding, high-pitched or weak cry, hypothermia, diaphoresis, or neonatal seizure activity. When left untreated, hypoglycemia can cause cerebral damage and mental retardation.

Clinical Therapy

Drug therapy. For at-risk infants who have not yet had a low blood sugar test, an oral feeding of 5% to 10% glucose or early breastfeeding is given with a follow-up blood glucose test within 30 to 60 minutes after feeding. If the baby cannot take oral glucose, a 5% to 10% glucose intravenous infusion is ordered at a rate that gives 6 to 8 mg/kg/min of glucose (at 90 to 100 mL/kg/day). For symptomatic acute hypoglycemia a bolus dose of $D_{10}W$ IV at a rate of 1 to 2 mL/kg is given followed by 5% to 10% glucose infusion. Alternative treatment may be administration of corticosteroid for prolonged cases of hypoglycemia. Intravenous glucose solution should be calculated based on body weight and fluid requirements and correlated with blood glucose tests to determine the adequacy of the infusion treatment.

Critical Nursing Assessments

1. Assess newborn and record for any risk factors.
   Be alert for special gestational newborns, such as premature, small for gestational age (SGA), and infant of diabetic mother (IDM) infants, and newborns with problems of asphyxia, cold stress, sepsis, or polycythemia who are particularly at risk. Also, maternal epidural anesthesia can alter maternal-fetal glucose homeostasis.

2. Assess blood glucose chemstrip on all newborns within 1 to 2 hours of birth (see Procedure: Performing a Heel Stick on a Newborn, on page 307). At-risk infants should be assessed no later than 2 hours after birth and before feedings, whenever there are abnormal signs, and then every 2 to 4 hours until stable.

3. Assess all newborns for symptoms of hypoglycemia.

Sample Nursing Diagnoses

- *Pain* related to multiple heel sticks for glucose monitoring.
- *Altered nutrition: less than body requirements* related to increased glucose use secondary to physiologic stresses.

- *Ineffective family coping* related to fear over infant's condition.

Critical Nursing Interventions

1. Based on agency glucose testing protocol, provide early feedings of breast milk or 5% to 10% glucose for infants at risk for hypoglycemia.

2. Obtain glucose oxidase reagent strip or optical bedside glucose analyzer reading per agency protocol. If <40 mg/dL, obtain STAT blood glucose per venous stick by lab. Then provide oral glucose water (about 1 oz) to infant. Recheck glucose oxidase reagent strip or optical bedside glucose analyzer reading in 1 hour. *Note:* If initial glucose oxidase reagent strip or optical bedside glucose analyzer reading is <20 mg/dL, obtain STAT blood glucose and prepare to start IV glucose therapy.

3. Monitor infants with low glucose levels who have been given oral glucose water for rebound hypoglycemia in approximately 3 to 4 hours.

4. If IV therapy is ordered by the physician or indicated by your agency protocol
   a. Start 5% to 10% dextrose and water IV on infusion pump on infants at risk for hypoglycemia and then continue glucose infusion as ordered.
   b. Administer infusion in peripheral vein of upper extremity to avoid lower extremity varicosities and potential tissue necrosis if IV infiltrates.
   c. Obtain glucose levels using glucose oxidase reagent strip or optical analyzer reading hourly during therapy per agency protocol. Obtain blood glucose levels q4–8hrs minimum.

5. Monitor titration of IV glucose during transition to oral glucose.

6. Provide comfort measures to ensure rest and maintain the optimal thermal environment specific for each newborn to reduce activity and glucose consumption.

Nonnutritive sucking may lower activity levels and conserve baby's energy levels.

7. Assist parents to identify feelings and concerns about baby's condition. Encourage and allow for maximum contact between parents and their baby.

8. Review the following critical aspects of the care you have provided:

   - Did I identify the baby's risk for hypoglycemia early in the baby's care?
   - Have I been alert for the early signs of hypoglycemia?
   - Have I monitored the blood glucose levels carefully and instituted care per agency protocol promptly?

Sample Nurse's Charting

0625 am T 97.7 °F, P 150, R 35. Ant. fontanelle soft & flat. Breath sounds equal bilaterally, slight substernal retractions. Abdomen soft and nondistended. Hypoactive bowel sounds. Fine tremors of arms and hands. Glucose reagent strips <40 mg/dL. Poor suck, took 25 mL of 5% G/W with difficulty. STAT lab blood glucose pending. Baby placed under radiant warmer to stabilize temperature. Dr. Rich notified of glucose level. M. Chin, RN

Evaluation

- Newborn's glucose level is stable at >40 mg/dL, and the baby is symptom free.
- Newborn is free from further complications.

Cold Stress

Overview

Cold stress occurs when babies are placed in an environment colder than their neutral thermal environment. When babies become chilled, they increase their oxygen consumption and use of glucose for physiologic processes. The complications that occur because of this alteration in metabolic processes are respiratory distress, respiratory and metabolic acidosis, hypoglycemia, and jaundice. Premature, SGA, hypoxic, hypoglycemic, and central nervous system (CNS) depressed newborns are at higher risk for becoming hypothermic and suffer the consequences.

Clinical Therapy

Initially, clinical management is directed to prevention and then to the management required by the specific complication.

Critical Nursing Assessments

1. Assess newborn temperature, using either axillary or skin probe method. *Be alert for* a drop in skin temperature (it drops before core temperature), which may be an early indicator of cold stress. *Tip:* Axillary temperature can be misleading because of the nearness to brown fat, which can increase heat production.
2. Assess for additional signs of hypothermia: shallow, irregular respirations; retractions; diminished reflexes; bradycardia; oliguria; and lethargy.
3. Assess for complications such as hyperbilirubinemia, hypoglycemia (blood glucose level <40 mg/dL), and respiratory distress.

Sample Nursing Diagnoses

- *Hypothermia* related to exposure to cold environment, trauma, illness, or inability to shiver.
- *Ineffective thermoregulation* related to immaturity.

Critical Nursing Interventions

1. Institute measures to prevent heat loss due to radiation, evaporation, convection, and conduction. Measures include the following: dry off baby immediately and remove wet linen after birth; place baby on prewarmed bed

under radiant heat source for all care and procedures; cover scales before weighing; warm stethoscope bell prior to auscultation; keep beds away from drafts and air vents; use warmed, humidified oxygen; keep baby wrapped when not skin to skin, cover head with stockinette hat, or place under radiant heat source with temperature probe in place; turn up thermostat in birthing area prior to birth; do not place warmer bed near windows or outside walls.

2. If chilled, rewarm slowly to prevent apnea (see Procedure: Thermoregulation of the Newborn, on page 321).

3. Monitor blood glucose levels for signs of hypoglycemia and arterial blood gases for signs of respiratory distress.

4. Carry out care needed by newborns placed under phototherapy to maintain stable temperature. (See the section on jaundice later in this chapter.)

5. Instruct parents about causes of temperature fluctuation, infant's current status, heat conservation methods, and temperature stabilization methods.

6. Observe parents as they take the newborn's temperature and determine that parents understand ways to minimize heat loss.

7. Review the following critical aspects of the care you have provided:
   - Have I provided for sufficient warmth during all procedures and care activities? During baths? During IV starts or blood work?
   - Have I been alert for any signs of hypoglycemia, hyperbilirubinemia, or respiratory distress?
   - Have I provided support and comfort to the baby?
   - Have I kept the parents informed?

Evaluation

- Baby is maintained in a neutral thermal environment.
- Parents understand the importance of preventing heat loss and methods to prevent complications of hypothermia.

Respiratory Distress Syndrome

Overview

Respiratory distress syndrome (RDS) is a condition associated with prematurity and any factor resulting in a deficiency of functioning surfactant, such as a diabetic mother or hypoxia. Clinical manifestations may present at birth or within a few hours after birth. Clinical manifestations are tachypnea, expiratory grunting, nasal flaring on inspiration, subcostal or intercostal retractions, pallor and cyanosis, apnea, labored breathing, increasing need for oxygen, and hypotonus. The chest x-ray shows diffuse reticulogranular density bilaterally, with portions of the air-filled tracheobronchial tree (air bronchogram) outlined by the opaque lungs. RDS usually resolves over 4 to 7 days unless surfactant replacement therapy has been used. A frequent complication is patent ductus arteriosus.

Clinical Therapy

Supportive management involves oxygen administration, ventilation therapy, blood gas studies to monitor oxygen and carbon dioxide levels, transcutaneous or pulse oximeter methods, and correction of acid-base imbalance. Ventilatory therapy is aimed at preventing hypoventilation and hypoxia. The degree of ventilatory support needed ranges from increasing oxygen concentration to the use of continuous positive airway pressure (CPAP) to intubation and full mechanical ventilation. Surfactant-replacement therapy has been shown to improve oxygenation rapidly and decrease the need for ventilatory support. Surfactant-replacement therapy must be administered by specially trained personnel.

Critical Nursing Assessment

1. Assess newborn for any risk factors. *Be alert for* premature infants and any infant suspected of hypoxia in utero or soon after birth.

2. Assess newborn's respiratory effort. Note chest wall movement, respiratory effort (grunting, nasal flaring, retractions), and color (cyanosis, pallor, duskiness) of skin

and mucous membranes; auscultate lung for bilateral air entry. *Tip:* At about 48 to 72 hours (if no surfactant-replacement therapy is given), when the alveoli begin to open up, watch the chest movement carefully, because the infant is at greatest risk for pneumothorax at this time.

3. Assess need for increased oxygen and assisted ventilation measures. *Note:* Normal PaO_2: 50–70 mm Hg, $PaCO_2$: 35–45 mm Hg, and pH 7.35–7.45. Monitor blood pressure (average for term infant, 80/45–40; preterm infant, 64/39).

4. Assess intake and output (I&O) and electrolytes. Increased labored breathing (work of breathing) causes an increase in insensible water losses. *Tip:* As the lungs open up, there is usually an increase in voiding because more fluid moves into the bloodstream to be excreted by the kidneys.

5. Assess for signs of infection: temperature instability, lethargy, poor feeding, and hypotonia.

Sample Nursing Diagnoses

- *Impaired gas exchange* related to inadequate lung surfactant.
- *Risk for infection* related to invasive procedures.
- *Ineffective thermoregulation* related to increased respiratory effort secondary to RDS.

Critical Nursing Interventions

1. Administer warmed, humidified oxygen by designated route: oxygen hood, continuous positive airway pressure (CPAP), and intubation (Figure 6–1).

2. Alter oxygen concentrations by 5% to 10% increments or per order to maintain adequate PaO_2 levels. Obtain blood gas levels after any significant change in oxygen concentration.

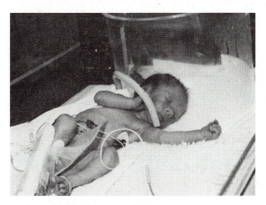

Figure 6–1   Infant in oxygen hood.

3. Obtain arterial blood gases per order. Maintain stable environment prior to blood gas studies (do not suction, change oxygen levels or ventilator settings, or disturb baby).

4. Suction as necessary. Secretions are sparse until second or third day, when the lungs start opening up. Watch transcutaneous oxygen monitor or pulse oximeter for desaturation during procedure.

5. Check and calibrate all monitoring and measuring devices every 8 hours.

6. Maintain patency of IVs.

7. Maintain a neutral thermal environment. Temperature instability increases oxygen consumption and metabolic acidosis.

8. Administer medications per order: antibiotics, diuretics, sedatives, and analgesics. Fentanyl and morphine are used for their analgesic and sedative effects. The use of pancuronium (Pavulon) for muscle relaxation is controversial.

9. Careful handwashing, use of gloves during procedures, and attention to infection control are essential.

10. Provide time to answer parents' questions about the baby's status and the equipment used and to give emotional support. Explain developmental supportive care to the parents.

11. Record and report all clinical observations.

Evaluation

- The risk of RDS is promptly identified, and early intervention is initiated.

- The newborn is free of respiratory distress and metabolic alterations.

- The parents verbalize their concerns about their baby's health problem and survival and understand the rationale behind management of their newborn.

Special Newborns and Their Associated Clinical Problems

Small for Gestational Age (SGA)

Physical Characteristics	Clinical Problems
Large-appearing head in proportion to chest and abdomen	1. **Perinatal asphyxia.** Chronic hypoxia in utero leaves little reserve to withstand the demands of labor and birth. Thus, intrauterine asphyxia occurs, with its potential systemic problems.
Loose, dry skin	
Scarcity of subcutaneous fat, with emaciated appearance	2. **Aspiration syndromes.** Gasping secondary to in utero hypoxia can cause aspiration of amniotic fluid into the lower airways or can lead to relaxation of the anal sphincter
Long, thin appearance	

Physical Characteristics

Sunken abdomen

Sparse scalp hair

Anterior fontanelle may be depressed

May have vigorous cry and appears alert

Birth weight below 10th percentile

Clinical Problems

with passage of meconium. This results in meconium aspiration with first breaths after birth.

3. **Heat loss.** Decreased ability to conserve heat results from diminished subcutaneous fat (used for survival in utero), depletion of brown fat in utero, and large surface area. The surface area is diminished somewhat because of the flexed position assumed by the SGA infant. (See "Cold Stress," discussed earlier in this chapter.)

4. **Hypoglycemia.** High metabolic rate (secondary to heat loss), poor liver glycogen stores, and inhibited gluconeogenesis lead to low blood sugar levels. (See "Hypoglycemia," discussed earlier in this chapter.)

5. **Hypocalcemia.** Calcium depletion secondary to birth asphyxia.

6. **Polycythemia.** A physiologic response to in utero chronic hypoxic stress.

Large for Gestational Age (LGA), especially Infant of Diabetic Mother (IDM)

Physical Characteristics

Appears fat and enlarged

If IDM, cushingnoid facial (round face) and neck features

Clinical Problems

1. **Hypoglycemia.** After birth the most common problem of an IDM is hypoglycemia. Even though the high maternal blood supply is lost, this newborn continues to produce high levels of insulin, which deplete

Physical Characteristics	Clinical Problems

Physical Characteristics

Overall ruddiness

Has enlarged liver, spleen, and heart

Initially lethargic then irritable and jittery

Clinical Problems

the blood glucose within hours after birth. IDMs also have less ability to release glucagon and catecholamines, which normally stimulate glucagon breakdown and glucose release. (See "Hypoglycemia," discussed earlier in this chapter.)

2. **Hypocalcemia.** Associated with prematurity and hyperphosphatemia or asphyxia.

3. **Hyperbilirubinemia.** This condition may be seen at 48 to 72 hours after birth. It may be caused by slightly decreased extracellular fluid volume, which increases the hematocrit level. Cephalhematoma, or enclosed hemorrhages, resulting from complicated vaginal birth may also cause hyperbilirubinemia. There may also be an increase in rate of bilirubin production in the presence of polycythemia. (See "Jaundice," discussed later in this chapter.)

4. **Polycythemia.** This condition may be caused by the decreased extracellular volume in IDMs. For IDMs hemoglobin A_{1c} binds oxygen, which decreases the oxygen available to the fetal tissues. This tissue hypoxia stimulates increased erythropoietin production, which increases the hematocrit level. (See "Polycythemia," discussed later in this chapter.)

Physical Characteristics	Clinical Problems

5. **Birth trauma,** such as fractures of the clavicle, facial nerve paralysis, Erb's paralysis, and diaphragmatic paralysis.

6. **Respiratory distress.** This complication occurs especially in newborns of White's classes A–C diabetic mothers. The composition of the phospholipids themselves is altered in the lungs of IDMs. (See "Respiratory Distress Syndrome," discussed earlier in this chapter.)

Preterm Infant

Physical Characteristics

Color—usually pink or ruddy but may be acrocyanotic; observe for cyanosis, jaundice, pallor, or plethora

Skin—reddened, translucent, blood vessels readily apparent, lack of subcutaneous fat

Lanugo—plentiful, widely distributed

Head size—appears large in relation to body

Clinical Problems

1. **Apnea of Prematurity.** Cessation of breathing for 20 seconds or longer or for less than 20 seconds when associated with cyanosis and bradycardia. It is thought to be primarily a result of neuronal immaturity, a factor that contributes to the tendency for irregular breathing patterns in preterm infants. Gastroesophageal reflux (GER) has been implicated in the production of apnea (causing laryngospasm).

2. **Patent ductus arteriosus.** Failure of ductus arteriosus to close because of decreased pulmonary arteriole musculature and hypoxemia.

3. **Respiratory distress syndrome (RDS).** Respiratory distress results

Physical Characteristics	**Clinical Problems**

Physical Characteristics

Skull—bones pliable, fontanelle smooth and flat

Ears—minimal cartilage, pliable, folded over

Nails—soft, short

Genitals—small; testes may not be descended

Resting position— flaccid, froglike

Cry—weak, feeble

Reflexes—poor sucking, swallowing, and gagging

Activity— jerky, generalized movements (seizure activity is abnormal)

Clinical Problems

from inadequate surfactant production. (See "Respiratory Distress Syndrome," discussed earlier in this chapter.)

4. **Intraventricular hemorrhage.** Up to 35 weeks' gestation the preterm infant's brain ventricles are lined by the germinal matrix, which is highly susceptible to hypoxic events. The germinal matrix is very vascular, and these blood vessels rupture in the presence of hypoxia.

5. **Hypocalcemia.** The preterm infant lacks adequate amounts of calcium secondary to early birth and growth needs.

6. **Hypoglycemia.** The preterm infant's decreased brown fat and glycogen stores and increased metabolic needs predispose this infant to hypoglycemia. (See "Hypoglycemia" and "Cold Stress," discussed earlier in this chapter.)

7. **Anemia of Prematurity.** The preterm infant is at risk for anemia because of the rapid rate of growth required, shorter red blood cell life, excessive blood sampling, decreased iron stores, and deficiency of vitamin E.

8. **Hyperbilirubinemia.** Immature hepatic enzymatic function decreases conjugation of bilirubin, resulting in increased bilirubin levels. (See "Jaundice," discussed later in this chapter.)

Physical Characteristics	**Clinical Problems**

9. **Infection.** The preterm infant is more susceptible to infection than the term infant. Most of the neonate's immunity is acquired in the last trimester. Therefore the preterm infant has decreased antibodies available for protection.

Postterm Infant

Physical Characteristics	**Clinical Problems**

Generally has normal size skull, but small body makes skull look large

Dry, cracked skin

Nails extending beyond fingertips

Profuse scalp hair

Subcutaneous fat layers depleted, leaving skin loose and giving an "old person" appearance

Long and thin body contour

Absent vernix

Often meconium staining (golden yellow to green) of skin, nails, and cord

1. **Hypoglycemia.** Nutritional deprivation and resultant depleted glycogen stores. (See "Hypoglycemia," discussed earlier in this chapter.)

2. **Meconium aspiration.** Response to hypoxia in utero.

3. **Polycythemia.** Due to increased production of red blood cells (RBCs) in response to hypoxia. (See "Polycythemia," discussed later in this chapter.)

4. **Congenital anomalies of unknown cause.**

5. **Seizure.** Due to hypoxic insult.

6. **Cold stress.** Due to loss or poor development of subcutaneous fat. (See "Cold Stress," discussed earlier in this chapter.)

Physical Characteristics

May have an alert, wide-eyed appearance symptomatic of chronic intrauterine hypoxia

Hematologic Problems of the Newborn

Anemia

Term (Hb <14 g/dL) Preterm (Hb <13 g/dL)

Characteristics

Pale, 3-second capillary refill, slow weight gain in first months of life. Tachycardia may be present. Profound tachycardia (HR >160) seen in hemorrhage.

Critical Nursing Management

Preventive: Term baby: Provide iron-fortified formula.
Preterm baby: May be given recombinant human erythropoietin (rEPO) and supplemental iron.

After 2 months of age switch to iron supplementation in formula.

Symptomatic newborn: (Needs increased oxygen, as do growing premature infants.) Administer packed RBCs transfusion:

- Warm blood.
- Give ordered amount over >30 minutes.
- Monitor for hypocalcemia and hypoglycemia.
- Do not exceed 10 mL/kg (of weight) volume per transfusion.
- Recheck Hct/Hb per agency protocol.

Polycythemia

Central venous Hct >65% and increased viscosity lead to impaired blood flow through blood vessels and decreased oxygen transport. LGA, IDM, SGA, and infants of pregnancy-induced hypertension (PIH) mothers are at risk.

Characteristics

Plethoric but cyanotic when crying. Tachypnea, tachycardia, possible murmur, congenital heart failure (CHF), respiratory distress. Feeding intolerance.

Hypoglycemia, lethargy, tremors, hypotonia, poor reflexes, and possible seizures secondary to decreased cerebral perfusion. Jaundice secondary to increased RBC breakdown. Microthrombi may occur in renal and cerebral artery.

Critical Nursing Management

Monitor pulse, respirations. Keep urine specific gravity <1.015.

Assess color at rest and when crying.

Obtain capillary blood sample for Hct (warm heel prior to heel stick; this increases blood flow and mirrors central Hct).

If heel stick Hct is >65%, obtain central Hct to verify polycythemia.

If Hct >65% but baby is asymptomatic: Increase fluid intake by 20–40 mL/kg/day. Recheck heel stick Hct q6h.

If Hct >65% and baby is symptomatic: Assist with partial exchange transfusion (remove some RBCs and replace with fresh frozen plasma [FFP] or 5% albumin, or plasmanate). The goal is to lower central venous Hct to 50 to 55%.

Monitor newborn's response to the procedure: Take VS *Be alert for* increased pulse, respiration rate, and temperature; signs of hypoglycemia. Obtain serial Hcts after exchange as ordered.

Jaundice

Overview

Hyperbilirubinemia is an above normal amount of bilirubin in the blood, which, when the level is high enough, produces jaundice. Jaundice can be seen as a visible yellowing of the skin, mucosa, sclera, and urine. **Physiologic jaundice** is the rise and fall in the serum bilirubin (indirect) level (4 to 12 mg/dL) by the fourth day after birth and peaking by the third to fifth day. Physiologic jaundice is common in term infants and is a result of neonatal hepatic immaturity. **Pathologic jaundice** is marked by yellow skin discoloration and an increase in the serum bilirubin level above 12.9 mg/dL in term infants and 15 mg/dL in preterm infants within 24 hours after birth. The bilirubin level rises faster than 5 mg/dL in 24 hours and may continue beyond a week in full-term newborns and 2 weeks in premature infants. Pathologic jaundice is most commonly associated with blood type or blood group incompatibility, infection, or biliary, hepatic, or metabolic abnormalities.

Clinical Therapy

Phototherapy and exchange transfusions are the primary medical treatments for hyperbilirubinemia. Phototherapy can be provided through conventional banks of phototherapy lights, by a fiber-optic blanket attached to a halogen light source around the trunk of the newborn, or by a combination of both delivery methods. Drug therapy (albumin, phenobarbital) may also be used.

Critical Nursing Assessments

1. Assess for risk factors.

   Be alert for prenatal history of Rh immunization; ABO incompatibility; maternal use of aspirin, sulfonamides, or antimicrobial drugs; Native American, Japanese, Chinese, or Korean nationality (predisposed to higher bilirubin levels); and yellow amniotic fluid, which indicates significant hemolytic disease.

2. Assess color of skin, sclera, and mucous membranes.

   Assessment technique: Observe in the daylight, or, using white fluorescent lights, blanch skin over bony prominence to remove capillary coloration and then assess degree of yellow discoloration. Assess oral mucosa and conjunctival sac in dark-skinned infants.

   Be alert for jaundice. In the first 24 hours after birth, it mandates immediate investigation. Pallor is associated with hemolytic anemia.

3. Assess laboratory results.

   Be alert for serum bilirubin increase of 5 mg/dL/day or more than 0.5 mg/hr, which indicates severe hemolysis or a pathologic process. Increased reticulocytes and decreased Hct and Hgb levels are also significant.

4. Assess clinical signs and symptoms.

   Be alert for poor feeding, lethargy, tremors, high-pitched cry, and absent Moro reflex; these are often the first signs of bilirubin encephalopathy (kernicterus). Vomiting, irritability, rigid musculature, opisthotonos, and seizures are later signs of encephalopathy and may indicate permanent damage.

Sample Nursing Diagnoses

- *Fluid volume deficit* related to decreased intake, loose stools, and increased insensible water loss.
- *Altered parenting* related to interruption in bonding between infant and parents secondary to separation.

Critical Nursing Interventions

Initiate feedings as soon as possible and continue q2–4 hours. While under phototherapy

1. Place infant under phototherapy lights unclothed, except perhaps for covering of genitals, to maximize exposure to lights. Phototherapy reduces bilirubin in the skin.

2. Cover infant's eyes when under the lights. Remove eye covers once a shift with phototherapy lights off. Inspect

eyes for pressure areas and conjunctivitis. Patches are removed to allow eye contact and facilitate parent-newborn interaction. Change eye patches every 24 hours. Mark patches with time, date, and right and left eye designation (to avoid cross contamination). Inspect eyes and check under the eye dressings for pressure areas.

Be alert for high-density light, which may cause retinal injury and corneal burns. Irritation from patches may cause corneal abrasions and conjunctivitis.

3. Monitor vital signs every 4 hours. If hypothermia or hyperthermia occurs, check temperature every hour.

4. Monitor intake and output every 8 hours. Weigh infant daily (provides accurate determination of fluid intake and insensible water loss caused by phototherapy). Determine urine specific gravities q8h. Notify physician if specific gravity >1.015, an indication of dehydration.

   Be alert for urine specific gravity results influenced by sugar, protein, blood, and urobiligen in the urine. Urine may be green because of the photodegradation of bilirubin. Stools are usually loose and green in color.

5. Provide fluid intake 25% above normal requirements to meet increase in insensible water losses and losses in the stools. Offer D_5W orally between breastfeeding or formula intake.

6. Reposition infant at least every 2 hours. Monitor skin for excoriations, rash, or bronzing of the skin. Change diaper and clean area as soon after stooling as possible to prevent skin breakdown.

   Tip: Ongoing assessment of skin must be done with the phototherapy lights off.

7. Turn phototherapy lights off when parents visit and for feedings. Coordinate care activities with parent visits so that parents have maximum contact with their baby with the phototherapy lights off.

8. Monitor phototherapy lights' wavelength using bilimeter every shift.

9. Monitor bilirubin levels every 8 hours for first 1 to 2 days or per agency protocol after discontinuation of phototherapy. Turn lights off when doing bilirubin laboratory tests. Bilirubin levels may rebound following phototherapy.

With the fiber-optic blanket, the light stays on at all times and the newborn is accessible for care, feeding, and diaper changes. The eyes are not covered. Fluid and weight loss are not complications of this system. Furthermore, the infant is accessible to the parents and the therapy is less alarming to parents than standard phototherapy. A combination of a fiber-optic light source in the mattress under the baby and a standard light source above has been recommended.

Evaluation

- The risks for development of hyperbilirubinemia are identified, and action is taken to minimize the potential impact of hyperbilirubinemia.
- The baby will not have any corneal irritation or drainage, skin breakdown, or major fluctuations in temperature.
- Parents will understand the rationale for, goal of, and expected outcome of therapy. Parents will verbalize their concerns about their baby's condition and identify how they can facilitate their baby's improvement.

Home Care

Continuing care of the family with a baby experiencing jaundice is important. The nurse will assess the family's status and information needs. Assessments of the baby will include color, temperature, fluid status, intake, number of voidings per day, and a pattern of bowel elimination. Behavioral assessment is important because the baby has spent time under phototherapy, which may have interfered with normal newborn-parent interaction. If phototherapy lights are being used, parents must agree that the baby will be exposed to the lights for long periods of time; that they will hold the baby for only short periods for feedings, comforting, and cleansing of the perineal area; and that the room temperature will be regulated to minimize heat loss. Fiber-optic phototherapy blankets eliminate the need for eye patches, decrease heat loss because the baby is clothed, and provide more opportunities for interaction between the baby and parents. The best method of home phototherapy depends on the cause of the hyperbilirubinemia and the rate of progression of the jaundice. The nurse can assist the parents in identifying and maximizing time for interaction.

Nursing Care Needs of Newborns of Substance-Abuse Mothers

Fetal Alcohol Syndrome (FAS)

Physical Characteristics	Early Neonatal Nursing Interventions
SGA	Monitor vital signs. *Be alert for* apnea, cyanosis, and hypothermia.
Abnormal features: microcephaly, craniofacial abnormalities, postnatal growth defects, congenital heart defects, mental retardation	Provide heat conservation measures (eg, cap for head, double wrap); for additional management see "Cold Stress," discussed earlier in this chapter.
	Note feeding problems/patterns (offer small, frequent feedings).
Withdrawal symptoms: hyperactivity, tremors, lethargy, poor suck reflex, exaggerated mouthing behaviors	Measure abdominal girth. Be alert for abdominal distention.
	Provide oxygen via nasal cannula or mask and bulb suction as ordered for respiratory distress or aspiration.
Can start after birth and persist throughout first month of life or longer	Place baby in dimly lit environment to prevent overstimulation.
	Observe for seizure activity.

Newborn of Drug-Dependent Mother

Physical Characteristics

SGA or premature

Withdrawal symptoms: nasal stuffiness, sneezing, yawning, increased sucking efforts

Increased secretions, difficulty feeding,

drooling, gagging, vomiting, diarrhea

Increased respiratory rate, incessant cry, respiratory distress

Irritability, tremors, hyperactivity, hypertonia, hyperreflexia, increased Moro reflex, disturbed sleeping pattern

Seizures (infrequent, but may occur in severe cases or with intrauterine asphyxia)

Fever, flushing, diaphoresis

Dehydration

Early Neonatal Nursing Interventions

Assess ability to feed (hyperactivity and increased secretions cause difficulty). *Be alert for* difficult feeder with poor suck and regurgitation/vomiting. Provide small, frequent feedings.

Position on side with head elevated to prevent choking.

Note frequency of diarrhea and vomiting and weigh every 8 hours during withdrawal.

Initiate safety precautions to prevent baby self-injury during periods of hyperactivity. Observe for seizures.

Decrease stimulating activities and provide quiet environment during withdrawal period. Provide gentle handling, pacifier, talk in soothing voice, play quiet music, swaddle snugly with hands near mouth, and hold as much as baby tolerates.

Encourage parent-infant attachment by explaining baby's behavior and giving comfort suggestions.

Administer drugs—phenobarbital, paragoric—as ordered for relief of withdrawal symptoms. Methadone should not be given because of possible newborn addiction to it.

Congenital Heart Disease in the Newborn Period

Overview

Congenital heart disease (CHD) occurs in about 4 to 5 per 1000 live births. The CHDs seen most often in the first week of life are transposition of the great vessels and hypoplastic left heart syndrome. Within the first month of life, the presenting conditions are coarctation of the aorta, ventricular septal defect, tetralogy of Fallot, and patent ductus arteriosus. Initial assessment of the newborn suspected of having CHD includes complete physical exam, blood pressure in all four extremities, electrocardiogram (ECG), chest x-ray, and evaluation of oxygenation in 100% oxygen. Now many newborns with congenital heart disease are diagnosed by fetal echocardiography, and corrective management can be done during the first month of life.

Clinical Therapy

Cardiac defects of the early newborn period include the following:

Patent Ductus Arteriosus (PDA)

↑ in females, maternal rubella, RDS, <1500 g preterm newborns, high-altitude births

Clinical Findings	Medical/Surgical Management
Harsh grade 2–3 machinery murmur at upper left sternal border (LSB) just beneath clavicle	Indomethacin—0.2 mg/kg orally (prostaglandin inhibitor).
	Surgical ligation or coils
↑ difference between systolic and diastolic pulse pressure	Use of O_2 therapy and blood transfusion to improve tissue oxygenation and perfusion
	Fluid restriction and diuretics

Clinical Findings

Medical/Surgical Management

Can lead to right heart failure and pulmonary congestion

↑ left atrial (LA) and left ventricular (LV) enlargement, dilated ascending aorta

↑ pulmonary vascularity

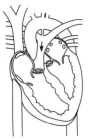

Patent ductus arteriosus.

Coarctation of Aorta

Can be preductal or postductal

Clinical Findings

Medical/Surgical Management

Absent or diminished femoral pulses

Increased brachial pulses

Late systolic murmur in left intrascapular area

Systolic BP in lower extremities

Enlarged left ventricle

Can present in CHF at 7–21 days of life

Surgical resection of narrowed portion of aorta

Prostaglandin E_1 to maintain peripheral perfusion

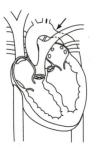

Coarctation of the aorta.

Transposition of Great Vessels (TGA)

($\uparrow$ females, IDMs, LGAs)

Clinical Findings	Medical/Surgical Management
Cyanosis at birth or within 3 days	Prostaglandin E_1 to vasodilate ductus to keep it open
Possible pulmonic stenosis murmur	Inotropie support
Right ventricular hypertrophy	Initial surgery to create opening between right and left side of heart if none exists
Polycythemia	Total surgical repair—usually the arterial switch done within first few days of life
"Egg on its side" x-ray	

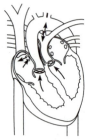

Complete transposition of great vessels. (All illustrations from *Congenital Heart Abnormalities.* Clinical Education Aid no. 7. Ross Laboratories, Columbus, Ohio.)

Hypoplastic Left Heart Syndrome

Clinical Findings	Medical/Surgical Management
Normal at birth—cyanosis and shocklike congestive heart failure develop within a few hours to days	Currently no effective corrective treatment (total repair)
	Palliative use of prostaglandin E_1
	Transplant
Soft systolic murmur just left of the sternum	

Clinical Findings	**Medical/Surgical Management**
Diminished pulses	
Aortic and/or mitral atresia	
Tiny, thick-walled left ventricle	
Large, dilated, hypertrophied right ventricle	
X-ray: cardiac enlargement and pulmonary venous congestion	

Critical Nursing Assessments

Nursing assessment of the following signs and symptoms assists in identifying the newborn with a cardiac problem:

1. Tachypnea: reflects increased pulmonary blood flow.
2. Dyspnea: caused by increased pulmonary venous pressure and blood flow; can also cause chest retractions, wheezing.
3. Color: ashen, gray, or cyanotic.
4. Difficulty in feeding: requires many rest periods before finishing even 1 or 2 oz.
5. Diaphoresis: beads of perspiration over the upper lip and forehead; may accompany feeding fatigue.
6. Stridor or choking spells.
7. Failure to gain weight.
8. Heart murmur: may not be heard in left-to-right shunting defects because the pulmonary pressure in the newborn is greater than pressure in the left side of the heart in the early newborn period.
9. Hepatomegaly: in right-sided heart failure, caused by venous congestion in the liver.

10. Tachycardia: pulse over 160, may be as high as 200.
11. Cardiac enlargement.

Critical Nursing Interventions

1. Give small, frequent feedings (oral) or gastric tube feeding to conserve energy (see Procedure: Performing Gavage Feeding, on page 315).
2. Obtain daily weights and strict intake and output.
   Be alert for failure to gain weight, inability to take more than an ounce of formula in 30 to 45 minutes of feeding, and decrease in urine output. Also note weight gain reflected as body edema.
3. Provide oxygen to relieve respiratory distress. Oxygen will not remove cyanosis.
4. Administer digoxin per order. Dosage should be double-checked by a second RN. It is given only after listening to the apical pulse for 1 minute and if no irregularities or slowing is noted. *Tip:* In most agencies, if pulse is lower than 120 bpm, check with physician before giving medication.
5. Diuretics (such as furosemide) are administered; potassium levels should be monitored because diuretics cause excretion of potassium.
6. Morphine sulfate, 0.05 mg/kg of body weight per dose, may be given for irritability. It decreases peripheral and pulmonary resistance and therefore decreases tachypnea. Place in semi-Fowler's position to ease breathing.
7. Fentanyl provides good pain control without respiratory depression seen with morphine sulfate.
8. Counsel parents on home care: administration of drugs, indications of drug toxicity, and measures used to prevent fatigue and promote nutrition for growth and development.

Evaluation

- Newborn's oxygen consumption and energy expenditure are minimal while at rest and during feedings.

- Newborn is protected from additional stresses such as infection, cold stress, and dehydration.
- Parents verbalize their concerns about their baby's health maintenance and need for ongoing follow-up care.

Congenital Anomalies: Identification and Care in Newborn Period

Congenital Hydrocephalus (1 in 1200 live births)

Nursing Assessments	Nursing Goals and Interventions
Enlarged head	Assess presence of hydrocephalus: Measure and plot occipital-frontal baseline measurements, then measure head circumference once a day.
Enlarged or full fontanelles	
Split or widened sutures	
"Setting sun" eyes	Check fontanelle for bulging and sutures for widening.
Head circumference >90% on growth chart	Assist with head ultrasound and transillumination.
	Maintain skin integrity: change position frequently.
	Use sheepskin pillow under head.
	Watch for signs of infection.

Choanal Atresia

Nursing Assessments	Nursing Goals and Interventions
Occlusion of posterior nares	Assess patency of nares: listen for breath sounds while holding baby's mouth closed and alternately compressing each nostril.
Cyanosis and retractions at rest	
Snorting respirations	Assist with passing feeding tube to confirm diagnosis.

Nursing Assessments	Nursing Goals and Interventions
Difficulty breathing during feeding	Maintain respiratory function: assist with taping airway in mouth to prevent respiratory distress.
Obstruction by thick mucus	Position with head elevated to improve air exchange.

Cleft lip (1 in 850–1000 live births)

Nursing Assessments	Nursing Goals and Interventions
Unilateral or bilateral visible defect	Provide nutrition: feed with special nipple.
May involve external nares, nasal cartilage, nasal septum, and alveolar process	Burp frequently (increased tendency to swallow air and reflex vomiting).
Flattening or depression of midfacial contour	Clean cleft with sterile water (to prevent crusting on cleft prior to repair).
	Support parental coping: assist parents with grief over loss of idealized baby.
	Encourage verbalization of their feelings about visible defect.
	Provide role model in interacting with infant. (Parents internalize others' responses to their newborn.)

Cleft Palate (1 in 2500 live births)

Nursing Assessments	Nursing Goals and Interventions
Fissure connecting oral and nasal cavity	Prevent aspiration/infection: place prone or in side-lying position to facilitate drainage.
May involve uvula and soft palate	Suction nasopharyngeal cavity (to prevent aspiration or airway obstruction).
May extend forward to nostril, involving	

Nursing Assessments	Nursing Goals and Interventions
hard palate and maxillary alveolar ridge	During neonatal period, feed in upright position with head and chest tilted slightly backward (to aid swallowing and discourage aspiration).
Difficulty in sucking	
Expulsion of formula through nose	
	Provide nutrition: feed with special nipple.
	Burp after each ounce (tend to swallow large amounts of air).
	Clean mouth with water after feedings.
	Provide parental support: refer parents to community agencies and support groups. Encourage verbalization of frustrations as feeding process is long and frustrating.
	Praise all parental efforts.
	Encourage parents to seek prompt treatment for upper respiratory infection (URI) and teach them ways to decrease incidence of URI.

Tracheoesophageal Fistula (Type 3) (1 in 3500 live births)

Nursing Assessments	Nursing Goals and Interventions
History of maternal hydramnios	Maintain respiratory status.
	Prevent aspiration.
Excessive mucus secretions	Quickly assess patency before putting to breast in birth area.
Constant drooling	Withhold feeding until esophageal patency is determined.
Abdominal distention beginning soon after birth	

Nursing Assessments	Nursing Goals and Interventions
Periodic choking and cyanotic episodes	Place on low intermittent suction to control saliva and mucus (to prevent aspiration pneumonia).
Immediate regurgitation of feeding	Place in warmed, humidified Isolette (liquefies secretions, facilitating removal).
Clinical symptoms of aspiration pneumonia (tachypnea, retractions, rhonchi, decreased breath sounds, cyanotic spells)	Elevate head of bed 20 to 40 degrees (to prevent reflux of gastric juices).
	Keep quiet (crying causes air to pass through fistula and to distend intestines, causing respiratory embarrassment).
Failure to pass nasogastric tube (see Figure 6-2)	Maintain fluid and electrolyte balance: give fluids to replace esophageal drainage and maintain hydration.
	Provide parent education: explain staged repair: provision of gastrostomy and ligation of fistula, then repair of atresia.
	Keep parents informed; clarify and reinforce physician's explanations regarding malformation, surgical repair, pre- and postoperative care, and prognosis.
	Involve parents in care of infant and in planning for future; facilitate touch and eye contact (to dispel feelings of inadequacy, increase self-esteem and self-worth, and promote incorporation of infant into family).

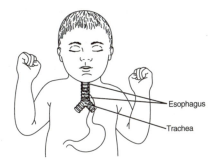

Figure 6–2 The most frequently seen type of congenital tracheoesophageal fistula and esophageal atresia.

Diaphragmatic Hernia (1 in 4000 live births)

Nursing Assessments

Difficulty initiating respirations

Gasping respirations with nasal flaring and chest retraction

Barrel chest and scaphoid abdomen

Asymmetric chest expansion

Breath sounds may be absent, usually on left side

Heart sounds displaced to right

Spasmodic attacks of cyanosis and difficulty in feeding

Bowel sounds may be heard in thoracic cavity

Nursing Goals and Interventions

Maintain respiratory status: immediately administer oxygen.

Never ventilate with a mask and bag and O_2 because stomach will inflate further, compressing the lungs.

Initiate gastric decompression.

Place in high semi-Fowler's position (to use gravity to keep abdominal organs' pressure off diaphragm).

Turn to affected side to allow unaffected lung expansion.

Carry out interventions to alleviate respiratory and metabolic acidosis.

Omphalocele (1 in 6000–10,000 live births)

Nursing Assessments	Nursing Goals and Interventions
Herniation of abdominal contents into base of umbilical cord	Maintain hydration and temperature: provide IV D_5LR and albumin for hypovolemia.
	Into base of umbilical cord
May have an enclosed transparent sac covering	May have an enclosed transparent sac covering
	Place infant in sterile bag up to above defect.
	Cover sac with moistened sterile gauze and place plastic wrap over dressing (to prevent rupture of sac and infection).
	Initiate gastric decompression by insertion of nasogastric tube attached to low suction (to prevent distention of lower bowel and impairment of blood flow).
	Prevent infection and trauma to defect.
	Position to prevent trauma to defect.
	Administer broad-spectrum antibiotics.

Myelomeningocele (0.5 in 1000 live births)

Nursing Assessments	Nursing Goals and Interventions
Saclike cyst containing meninges, spinal cord, and nerve roots in thoracic and/or lumbar area	Prevent trauma and infection.
	Position on abdomen or on side and restrain (to prevent pressure and trauma to sac).
	Meticulously clean buttocks and genitals after each voiding and

Nursing Assessments	**Nursing Goals and Interventions**
Myelomeningocele directly connects to subarachnoid space so hydrocephalus often occurs	defecation (to decrease possibility of infection).
	May put protective covering over sac (to prevent rupture and drying).
No response or varying response to sensation below level of sac	Observe sac for oozing of fluid or pus.
	Credé bladder (apply downward pressure on bladder with thumbs, moving urine toward the urethra) as ordered to prevent urinary stasis.
May have constant dribbling of urine	
Incontinence or retention of stool	Assess amount of sensation and movement below defect.
Anal opening may be flaccid	Observe for complications: obtain occipital-frontal circumference baseline measurements once a day (to detect hydrocephalus). Check fontanelle for bulging.
Assess anterior fontanelle for bulging	

Congenital Dislocated Hip (Developmental Dysplasia) (1 in 200 live births)

Nursing Assessments	**Nursing Goals and Interventions**
Asymmetric gluteal and anterior thigh fold	Maintain abduction position via Pavlik harness or plastic abduction splint.
One leg may be shorter	Provide perineal care to prevent skin breakdown.
Positive Ortolani test	Instruct parents on home care.

Clubfoot (1 in 1000 live births)

Nursing Assessments

Nursing Goals and Interventions

Abnormal turning of foot/feet either inward or outward

Unable to rotate to normal position

If casted, keep casts dry and protect legs from irritation. Carry out circulatory and neurologic checks.

Soothe infant during and after castings.

Provide parents with cast-care instructions (handling, cleaning, and signs of complications).

Imperforate Anus (1 in 5000 live births)

Nursing Assessments

Nursing Goals and Interventions

Visible anal membrane

Inability to take rectal temperature

No passage of meconium

Abdominal distention

Monitor for passage of first stool.

Measure abdominal girth (increasing abdominal distention).

Prepare parents for possible need for temporary colostomy.

Perinatally Acquired Newborn Infections

Group B Streptococcus

1% to 2% colonized, with 1 in 10 developing disease

Early onset—usually within hours of birth or within first week

Late onset—1 week to 3 months

Critical Nursing Assessments

Critical Nursing Interventions

Assess for risk factors (eg, low Apgar scores)

Assess for severe respiratory distress

Closely monitor VS for signs of respiratory distress and infection.

Critical Nursing Assessments

(grunting and cyanosis)

May become apneic or demonstrate symptoms of shock

Meconium-stained amniotic fluid seen at birth

Critical Nursing Interventions

Assist with x-ray—shows aspiration pneumonia or respiratory distress syndrome.

Immediately obtain blood, gastric aspirate, external ear canal, and nasopharynx cultures.

Administer antibiotics, usually aqueous penicillin or ampicillin combined with gentamicin as soon as cultures are obtained.

Initiate referral to evaluate for blindness, deafness, and learning or behavioral problems.

Gonorrhea

Approximately 30% to 35% of newborns born vaginally to infected mothers are infected. Onset 7 to 14 days after birth.

Critical Nursing Assessments

Assess for ophthalmia neonatorum (conjunctivitis)

Purulent discharge and corneal ulcerations

Neonatal sepsis with temperature instability, poor feeding response, and/or hypotonia, jaundice

Critical Nursing Interventions

Administer 1% silver nitrate solution or ophthalmic antibiotic ointment (see Drug Guide: Erythromycin Ophthalmic Ointment, on page 271), or, in lieu of silver nitrate, administer penicillin.

May give aqueous penicillin G IM as ordered if mother's culture positive.

Maintain body substance isolation during procedures, educate parents regarding need for careful hand washing, and so forth.

Initiate follow-up referral to evaluate any loss of vision.

Chlamydia Trachomatis

Acquired during passage through birth canal. Appears 5 to 14 days after birth.

Critical Nursing Assessments

Critical Nursing Interventions

Assess for perinatal history of preterm birth

Symptomatic newborns present with pneumonia— conjunctivitis (purulent yellow discharge and eyelid swelling) after 3 to 4 days

Chronic follicular conjunctivitis (corneal neovascularization and conjunctival scarring)

Instill ophthalmic erythromycin (see Drug Guide: Erythromycin Ophthalmic Ointment, on page 271).

Initiate follow-up referral for eye complications and late development of pneumonia at 4 to 11 weeks postnatally.

Herpes Type 2 (1 in 75,000 live births)

Usually transmitted during vaginal birth.

Critical Nursing Assessments

Critical Nursing Interventions

Assess for small cluster vesicular skin lesions over all the body

Check perinatal history for active herpes genital lesions

Disseminated form— DIC, pneumonia, hepatitis with jaundice,

Carry out careful handwashing and gown and glove isolation with linen precautions.

Administer intravenous vidarabine (Vira A) or acyclovir (Zovirax).

Initiate follow-up referral to evaluate potential sequelae of microcephaly, spasticity, seizures, deafness, or blindness.

Critical Nursing Assessments	Critical Nursing Interventions
hepatosplenomegaly, and neurologic abnormalities	Encourage parental rooming-in and touching of their newborn.
Without skin lesions, see fever or subnormal temperature, respiratory congestion, tachypnea, and tachycardia	Show parents appropriate handwashing procedures and precautions to be used at home if mother's lesions are active.
	Obtain throat, conjunctiva, cerebrospinal fluid (CSF), blood, urine, and lesion cultures to identify herpesvirus type 2 antibodies in serum IgM fraction.
	Cultures positive in 24 to 48 hours.

AIDS (placental transmission)

Critical Nursing Assessments	Critical Nursing Interventions
Assess mother for risk factors: HIV-positive, infected sexual partners, drug use, or needle sharing	Take vital signs q4h.
Assess for S & S of opportunistic infections, failure to thrive, weight loss, more than 3 diarrheal stools per day, feeding intolerance, oral candidiasis infection, diaper rash, hepatosplenomegaly, respiratory difficulty, lethargy, temperature instability, generalized	Provide meticulous skin care and change diaper after each voiding and stooling.
	Maintain standard precautions per agency.
	Provide small frequent feedings and food supplementation.
	Monitor stools for amount, type, consistency, change in patterns, occult blood, and reducing substances.
	Avoid giving infant any injections, drawing blood, or instilling eye medication until initial bath with mild soap and water. Wear disposable gloves.

Critical Nursing Assessments	Critical Nursing Interventions
skin rash, lymphadenopathy, and loss of developmental milestones	Instruct woman and family on newborn health needs and need for frequent position changes.
Assess skin for breakdown or rashes	Determine parental understanding of AIDS.
Assess cause of parental fear	Provide emotional support to mother and family if breastfeeding was desired.
	Provide list of contact persons for available community resources and information about current and experimental treatment.

Oral Candida Infection (Thrush)

Acquired during passage through birth canal.

Critical Nursing Assessments	Critical Nursing Interventions
Assess buccal mucosa, tongue, gums, and inside the cheeks for white plaques (seen at 5 to 7 days of age)	Differentiate white plaque areas from milk curds by using cotton tip applicator (if it is thrush, removal of white areas causes raw bleeding areas).
Check diaper area for bright-red, well-demarcated eruptions	Maintain cleanliness of hands, linen, clothing, diapers, and feeding apparatus.
Assess for thrush periodically when newborn is on long-term antibiotic therapy	Instruct breastfeeding mothers on treating their nipples with nystatin.
	Administer gentian violet (1% to 2%) swabbed on oral lesions 1 hour after feeding, or nystatin instilled in baby's oral cavity and on mucosa.
	Swab skin lesions with topical nystatin.

Critical Nursing Interventions

Discuss with parents that gentian violet stains mouth and clothing.

Avoid placing gentian violet on normal mucosa; causes irritation.

Chapter 7

The Postpartum Client

The period of time (approximately 6 weeks) following child-birth, during which the body returns to a prepregnant state, is called the **puerperium.** Because of current practice most women are discharged within 1-2 days. Nursing care during this time focuses on assessment for developing complications and on client teaching. The nurse should use every opportunity to explain the normal physiologic changes to the woman so that she will be able to recognize deviations and contact her care-giver if complications arise.

Postpartum Nursing Assessments

Table 7–1 identifies the basic assessments the postpartum nurse should make, explains postpartum physiologic changes, and identifies basic teaching that is indicated.

Nursing Interventions for Postpartum Discomfort

Perineal Discomfort: Episiotomy and Hemorrhoids

- During the first few hours after childbirth the woman can use an ice glove or chemical ice bag on the perineal area. If a glove is used, wash it first to remove powder, then wrap it in a washcloth or towel. Leave on 20 minutes, then off 10 minutes.

- After the first few hours the woman can take a sitz bath, usually ordered for 20 minutes tid or qid and prn. It is soothing and cleansing, and its warmth promotes healing.

  1. Some research suggests that a cool sitz bath may be more effective than a warm sitz bath in reducing

Table 7–1 Postpartum Assessment and Teaching

Physiologic Changes	Nursing Assessment	Client Teaching
Vital Signs		
Temperature: normal range; may increase to 100.4°F (38°C) because of exertion and mild dehydration.	Normal: 98–100.4°F [36.2–38°C]. After first 24 hours temperature > 100.4F (38°C) suggests infection.	Advise woman that following discharge, if she experiences chills, malaise, and so forth, she should take her temperature and report fever to her caregiver.
Pulse: puerperal bradycardia may occur for 6 to 10 days postpartum because of decreased blood volume and cardiac strain and increased stroke volume.	Pulse: 50–90 beats/min. Tachycardia may result from difficult labor and birth or from hemorrhage. Assess for additional signs of hemorrhage.	Explain that pulse slows normally. Advise woman to report palpitations, rapid pulse.
Respirations: unchanged.	Respirations normally 16–24/min. If decreased, evaluate for medication effects; if marked tachypnea present, assess for signs of pneumonia or other respiratory disease.	Advise woman to report symptoms of complications, including difficulty breathing, cough, rapid respirations.
Blood pressure (BP): remains consistent with baseline BP. A slight decrease may indicate normal physiologic readjustment to decreased intrapelvic pressure.	BP elevated: consider pregnancy-induced hypertension (PIH), especially if accompanied by headache (see Chapter 2). Note proteinuria, edema. BP decreased: evaluate for additional signs of hemorrhage (rapid pulse, clammy skin).	Explain findings to woman.

(Continued)

209

Table 7–1 Postpartum Assessment and Teaching (Continued)

Physiologic Changes	Nursing Assessment	Client Teaching
Breasts		
Immediately after birth, breasts are smooth, soft, and show changes in pigmentation, presence of striae, characteristic of pregnancy.	Assess fit and support provided by bra, which should hold all the breast tissue, and, for breastfeeding women, have cotton straps that do not stretch. Nursing bras have flaps that open for breastfeeding.	Discuss importance of wearing a well-fitting bra 24 hours a day until breast milk is suppressed in nonnursing mother or until breastfeeding mother stops nursing.
Anterior pituitary secretion of prolactin promotes milk production by stimulating alveolar cells of breast. Oxytocin, produced by posterior pituitary when infant suckles, promotes milk letdown reflex and flow of milk results. At this time breasts are producing colostrum, which is creamy and high in maternal antibodies. By 2 to 4 days after childbirth, the breast begins producing milk. Breasts tend to become full and hard due to milk production and venous congestion. This is called engorgement.	Assess size and shape of breasts (one breast often larger than the other). Palpate and note whether breast is soft (initially), somewhat firm (associated with filling), firm (full of milk), or hard (engorgement). Note tenderness, palpable mass, heat, and edema (suggest caked breast or mastitis). If present, assess for other signs of infection, including fever malaise. Assess nipples for fissures, cracks, soreness, inversion.	Discuss methods for relieving discomfort or engorgement for nonnursing and nursing mothers as indicated. (See "Breast Engorgement in the Nonnursing Mother" in this chapter, and Table 7–2.) Review signs of infection.

Abdomen

Abdominal wall is stretched; appears loose and flabby for some time. Tone can improve in 2 to 3 months with exercise. Diastasis recti abdominis is a separation of the rectus abdominis muscle so that a portion of abdominal wall has no muscular support.

Abdomen feels soft, may have a "doughy" texture.

Discuss exercises that can be done to improve tone. (See discussion on page 225 and Figure 7-3.)

Uterus

Involution: rapid reduction in size of the uterus and its return to a near prepregnant size following childbirth. Involution is enhanced by an uncomplicated birth, breastfeeding, and early ambulation. Immediately following expulsion of the placenta, uterus is contracted, about the size of a large grapefruit, located midway between symphysis and umbilicus. It gradually rises up to the level of the umbilicus as blood collects and forms clots within the uterus. It stays there for about 1 day,

See Procedure: Assessing the Fundus Following Vaginal Birth, on page 288 for correct technique. Fundus should be firm and in the midline. Displacement to the side may be caused by a full bladder. A fundus that is not firm is called "boggy." This may be caused by pressure from a full bladder, by the presence of clots, or because of diminished contractility in a woman who has borne several children. Massage fundus gently with the fingertips until firm; if the uterus does not contract, more vigorous massage may be

Teach mother to evaluate her fundus herself. If it is boggy she can then massage it until it is firm and report this to the nurse.
Explain the importance of voiding regularly to avoid pressure on the uterus.

(Continued)

211

Table 7–1 Postpartum Assessment and Teaching (*Continued*)

Physiologic Changes	Nursing Assessment	Client Teaching
then decreases in size about one finger breadth/day. Within 10 days to 2 weeks it is again a pelvic organ. Muscles stay contracted to clamp off blood vessels at placental site to prevent hemorrhage. Uterine ligaments are still stretched so uterus is movable and can be displaced by a full bladder. Placental site takes up to 6 weeks to heal. Healing occurs by exfoliation so that no scar is formed, which would limit area available for future placental implantation.	necessary; assess bladder for distention and have woman void if necessary. **Attempt to express clots only when the uterus is firm; do not attempt to express clots from a boggy uterus.** This could cause uterine inversion. If bogginess remains or returns, notify physician or nurse-midwife. Note height of uterus in relation to umbilicus and chart. Example: Uterus firm, in the midline 1 FB↑ U.	
Lochia After birth the uterus rids itself of the debris that remains by discharging lochia. **Lochia rubra**, which lasts for 2 to 3 days, is dark red, like menstrual flow. **Lochia serosa** lasts from about the 3rd to	Assess lochia for character, amount, odor (should have a slightly musty but not offensive odor, foul odor suggests infection), and the presence of clots. A few small clots are normal, but large	Instruct woman not to use tampons postpartum because of risk of infection. Perineal pads are generally used with a sanitary belt. (Adhesive-backed pads that are placed inside the panties move

10th day. It is similar to serosanguineous drainage. **Lochia alba**, the final discharge, is a creamy brownish or yellowish discharge. When it stops the cervix is considered closed and risk of ascending infection is decreased. Lochia tends to be more abundant on arising probably because of pooling in the vagina during the night). The amount may also increase with breastfeeding (oxytocin, released with suckling, stimulates uterine contraction) and with exertion. The type, amount, and consistency of lochia indicate the degree of healing of the placental site. Persistent lochia rubra or a return to rubra from serosa may indicate subinvolution or late postpartal hemorrhage.

Perineum

Following birth the soft tissue of the perineum may be edematous and bruised. Episiotomy may be present.

clots are abnormal and should be investigated. Flow should never exceed moderate amount (eg, four to eight perineal pads daily). If woman reports heavy bleeding, have woman apply clean pad and reassess in 1 hour. If she reports passage of clots, ask her to save all pads with clots and not flush toilet if clots are expelled with urination. If accurate assessment of blood loss is necessary, weigh pads after first balancing scale with a clean, dry pad; 1 g is considered equivalent to 1 mL blood. Chart amount, followed by character. Example: Lochia: small amount, rubra, no clots.

Perineum should appear intact; slight edema and bruising are normal. Marked fullness, bruising, and pain may indicate

more when the woman walks and may spread contamination from the anal area to the episiotomy and vaginal opening.) Many young woman have never worn a belt and may need assistance the first time. (Some agencies instead use a snug mesh panty that holds the pad in place.) Explain the progression of lochia from rubra to serosa to alba. Instruct the woman to save and report excessive clots and heavily saturated pads. She should also report failure of lochia to progress from rubra to serosa or a return to rubra from serosa. Teach woman to change pads with each voiding or bowel movement and after showering or use of a sitz bath.

The woman may apply an ice glove or pack initially to prevent edema. Teach woman to use a perineal bottle filled with

(Continued)

213

Table 7–1 Postpartum Assessment and Teaching *(Continued)*

Physiologic Changes	Nursing Assessment	Client Teaching
Woman may also have some hemorrhoids as a result of pushing during labor.	hematoma and require further evaluation. Inspect episiotomy. There should be no redness, edema, ecchymosis, or drainage, and the edges should be well approximated. If hemorrhoids are present, they should be small and nontender; full, reddened, inflamed hemorrhoids are painful and require comfort measures (see "Perineal Discomfort: Episiotomy and Hemorrhoids," in this chapter).	warm water or a surgigator after each voiding to wash the perineum and promote healing. Teach importance of wiping from the front (urinary meatus) to the back (anal area) to prevent contamination of the episiotomy from the anal area. Teach comfort measures for hemorrhoids.
Urinary Tract Urinary output greatly increases in the early postpartum period because of diuresis. Woman may have difficulty voiding because of decreased bladder sensation, swelling and bruising of tissues around urethra, increased bladder capacity, and difficulty voiding while recumbent.	Assess voiding; woman should be voiding sufficient quantities (at least 250–300 mL) every 4 to 6 hours; ask about symptoms of urinary tract infection (UTI) (urgency, frequency, dysuria); note whether bladder is palpable; determine whether fundus is in the midline. Palpate costovertebral angle (CVA) for tenderness.	Explain the importance of adequate voiding; help woman with difficulty by providing privacy, suggesting she pour warm water over perineum, encouraging ambulation, and describing visualization techniques. Identify symptoms of UTI; explain importance of adequate fluid intake (at least 2000 mL) daily.

Lower Extremities Stasis of blood in legs due to positioning, trauma to blood vessels, and use of stirrups increases risk of thrombophlebitis.	Inspect legs for redness edema. Assess for Homans' sign (pain in calf when foot sharply dorsiflexed); palpate for tenderness, warmth.	Stress the importance of early ambulation to promote venous return. Encourage woman to avoid crossing legs or using knee-gatch position on bed.
Bowel Elimination Bowels tend to be sluggish because of lingering effects of progesterone, decreased abdominal muscle tone, and lack of blood and fluid. Woman may fear bowel movement will be painful because of episiotomy or hemorrhoids.	Ask woman about bowel elimination. She should have a normal bowel movement by second or third day after birth. Stool softeners may be indicated if hemorrhoids or episiotomy increase possibility of discomfort.	Explain importance of bowel elimination. Encourage ambulation, increased fluid intake, diet high in roughage. Explain risks of constipation.

perineal edema. Offer women a choice of temperature.

2. **Procedure:** Disposable sitz tubs fit over a toilet with raised lid. At home the woman can fill a bathtub with 4 to 6 in. of water at a comfortable (not too hot) temperature. She should not bathe in the sitz tub water because of the risk of introducing infection.

3. Topical agents such as Dermoplast aerosol spray or Nupercainal ointment may be applied by the woman following a sitz bath.

- The previously described treatments are effective for episiotomy and hemorrhoids. In addition, suggested nursing interventions for hemorrhoids include the following:

1. Encourage side-lying position.

2. Teach the woman to reinsert hemorrhoids digitally. To do this she lies on her side, places lubricant on her finger, and applies steady gentle pressure against the hemorrhoids, pushing them inside. She should hold them in place for 1 to 2 minutes, then withdraw her finger. The anal sphincter should then hold them in place. She should maintain the side-lying position for a period of time.

3. Witch hazel pads may be placed against the hemorrhoids and held in place by the perineal pad. They are soothing and cool.

4. Encourage actions that help prevent constipation such as increased fluid intake, roughage in diet, early ambulation, and use of stool softeners as prescribed.

Afterpains

Afterpains are the result of intermittent uterine contractions and are more common in multiparas, women who had a multiple pregnancy, and women who had hydramnios. They may be intensified by breastfeeding because oxytocin is released when the baby suckles.

- Have woman lie prone with small pillow under abdomen. This places constant pressure on the uterus, causing it to remain contracted. Tell her the pain will be intensified for a few minutes but then will subside.
- Administer analgesic as needed. For breastfeeding women, administer about 1 hour before scheduled feeding.

Postpartum Diaphoresis

- Diaphoresis results as the body works to eliminate excess fluid and waste. It frequently occurs at night, and the woman awakens drenched with perspiration.
- Protect woman from chilling by changing bedding and providing a fresh gown.
- Encourage a shower (unless cultural practices forbid it).
- Prevent thirst by offering fluids as the woman desires.

Discomfort from Immobility

- The woman may have mild to severe muscular aches from pushing during the second stage and birth.
- Encourage early ambulation. The woman may be light-headed initially because of blood loss, fatigue, or medication, so assist her the first few times. This is especially important during the first shower, when heat may add to the problem.
- Stay close, have a call light and chair readily available, and check the woman frequently.

Suppression of Lactation in the Nonnursing Mother

- Lactation may be suppressed through mechanical inhibition, which includes the following:
  1. Have the woman wear a well-fitting, supportive bra continuously until lactation is suppressed (about 5 days). The bra is removed only for showers. A breast binder may be applied if the woman prefers or if no bra is available.

2. Apply ice packs over axillary area of both breasts for 20 minutes qid.

3. Avoid any stimulation of breasts by the woman, her partner, or her infant.

4. Avoid warmth, which stimulates milk production; avoid letting shower water flow over breasts.

Breast Engorgement in the Nonnursing Mother

- Interventions are the same as those for suppression.
- Administer analgesics as necessary.

  Note: Breast engorgement in the nursing mother is addressed in Chapter 9.

Infant Feeding

Breastfeeding

- Physiology of lactation:

  1. The hormone prolactin, from the anterior pituitary, is initially responsible for milk production.

  2. Oxytocin, from the posterior pituitary, is responsible for the letdown reflex, which triggers the flow of milk.

  3. The letdown reflex is stimulated by infant suckling, but it can also be stimulated by the newborn's presence or cry, or even thinking about the infant. It may also occur during sexual orgasm because oxytocin is released.

  4. The letdown reflex may be inhibited by a mother's lack of self-confidence, feelings of fear or embarrassment, or physical discomfort.

  5. Milk production is based on the law of supply and demand. Repeated inhibition of the letdown reflex or failure to empty the breasts completely and frequently may decrease milk supply.

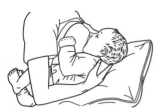

Football hold

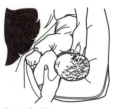

Lying down

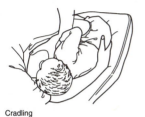

Cradling

Across the lap

Figure 7–1 Examples of breastfeeding position changes to facilitate thorough breast emptying and prevent nipple soreness.

- Breastfeeding technique:
  1. Put the newborn to breast as soon as possible.
  2. Position baby so that entire body is turned toward breast. Figure 7–1 shows a variety of positions.
  3. Direct nipple straight into infant's mouth with as much of the areola included as possible so that as infant sucks, his or her jaws compress the ducts under the areola, where milk is stored (see Figure 7–2). To do this, the mother holds the breast with her thumb placed on the upper portion and the remainder of her fingers cupping the breast. She then lightly strokes the infant's lips with the nipple.
  4. Avoid the temptation to use a nipple shield. This confuses the baby and makes it more difficult to learn to nurse.
  5. Avoid setting artificial time limits on the amount of time the baby should nurse. It may take up to

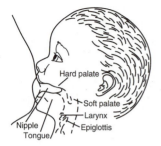

Labels on figure: Hard palate, Soft palate, Larynx, Epiglottis, Nipple, Tongue

Figure 7–2 To nurse effectively, it is important that the infant's mouth cover the majority of the areola to compress the ducts below. (Courtesy of Ross Laboratories, Columbus, Ohio.)

3 minutes for the letdown reflex to occur. Instead, advise the woman to let the baby nurse at one breast as long as the baby is sucking well and positioned correctly.

6. To avoid trauma to the breasts the mother should not let the infant sleep with the nipple in its mouth.

7. When the baby has emptied the first breast she or he is burped and switched to the second breast. (See discussion on burping on page 224.) When the baby has completed feeding she or he is burped again.

8. The baby's suck tends to be most vigorous initially. To avoid undue trauma to the breasts the mother should alternate the breast from which she nurses first.

9. Babies are obligatory nose breathers. To avoid having the breast block the nares, the mother should either lift the breast slightly or compress the breast tissue away from the baby's nose.

10. To prevent trauma to the nipple the mother should break suction before removing the infant from the breast by inserting a finger into the infant's mouth, next to the nipple.

11. When feeding is completed the woman should wash the nipples with warm water to prevent milk drying and should inspect them for trauma.

12. Frequent nursing helps establish a good supply of milk and prevents nipple trauma from the too vigorous suck of a ravenous infant. Thus, during the first few days the mother should nurse frequently (every 1 1/2 to 3 hours).

13. Table 7–2 identifies self-care measures a woman may use if she experiences common breastfeeding problems. See Chapter 9 for suggested interventions for other common problems.

Bottle Feeding

- Bottle feeding is also a nurturing choice for infant feeding and allows both parents to share in this nurturing activity with their child. A variety of commercial formulas are available.

- Whole milk and skim milk should not be used for children under 2 years. Whole milk has too high a protein content; skim milk also has too much protein and lacks adequate calories and essential fatty acids.

- Formula tends to be digested more slowly, so the bottle-fed infant may go longer between feedings. Infants are usually fed "on demand," which typically is every 3 to 5 hours.

- Bottle-feeding technique:

  1. The mother should assume a comfortable position with adequate arm support so that she can cradle her baby in her arm close to her body.

  2. The bottle should be held, not propped, with the baby's head somewhat elevated. Feeding the infant horizontally may result in positional otitis media.

  3. The nipple should have a large enough hole to permit milk to flow in drops when the bottle is inverted. Too large an opening may cause overfeeding and regurgitation.

  4. The nipple should be pointed directly into the mouth and on top of the tongue. It should be kept full of formula to avoid ingestion of extra air.

Table 7–2   Self-Care Measures for the Woman with Breastfeeding Problems

Nipple Inversion

Use Hoffman's exercises to increase protractility.

Use special breast shields such as Woolrich or Eschmann.

Use hand to shape nipple when beginning to nurse.

Apply ice for a few minutes prior to feeding to improve nipple erection.

Use electric or hand pump to cause nipple prominence, express a few drops of breast milk, then switch to regular nursing.

Inadequate Letdown

Massage breasts prior to nursing.

Feed in a quiet, private place, away from distraction.

Take a warm shower before nursing to relax and stimulate letdown.

Apply warm pack for 20 minutes before nursing.

Use relaxation techniques and focus on letdown.

Drink water, juice, or noncaffeinated beverages before and during feeding.

Avoid overfatigue by resting when the baby sleeps, feeding while lying down, and having quiet time alone.

Develop a conditioned response by establishing a routine for starting feedings.

Allow the baby sufficient time (at least 10–15 minutes per side) to trigger the letdown reflex.

Use breast-alternating method (either use different breast for each feeding or switch breasts several times during a single feeding).

If all else fails obtain a prescription for oxytocin nasal spray from the health care provider.

Nipple Soreness

Ensure that infant is correctly positioned at the breast with the infant's ear, shoulder, and hip in straight alignment.

Rotate breastfeeding positions.

Use finger to break suction before removing infant from the breast.

Hold baby close when feeding to avoid undue pulling on nipple.

Do not allow baby to sleep with nipple in mouth.

Nurse more frequently.

Begin nursing on less sore breast.

Apply ice to nipples and areola for a few minutes prior to feeding.

Protect nipples to prevent skin breakdown.

Clean nipple gently with warm water.

Allow nipples to air dry, dry nipples with hair dryer set on low heat, or expose nipples to sunlight initially for 30 seconds, then increase to 3 minutes.

Table 7–2   *(Continued)*

If clothing rubs nipples, use ventilated shields to keep clothing away from skin.

To promote healing, apply a small amount of breast milk to nipple and areola after nursing and allow to dry.

The routine application of ointment to nipple, areola, or breast (eg, lanolin, Massé cream, Eucerin cream, or A and D ointment) should be discouraged.

Apply tea bags soaked in warm water.

Change breast pads frequently.

Nurse long enough to empty breasts completely.

Alternate breasts several times during feedings.

Cracked Nipples

Use interventions discussed under sore nipples.

Inspect nipples carefully for cracks or fissures.

Temporarily stop nursing on the affected breast and hand express milk for a day or two until cracks heal.

Maintain healthy diet. Protein and vitamin C are essential for healing.

Use a mild p.o. analgesic such as acetaminophen for discomfort 20–30 minutes before feedings.

Consult health care providers if signs of infection develop.

Nipple shield should be tried before nursing on a breast is permanently discontinued, but it should be used only as a last resort. Some women find it contributes to their discomfort. Consult a lactation specialist prior to use.

Breast Engorgement

Nurse frequently (every 1½ to 3 hours) around the clock.

Wear a well-fitting, supportive bra at all times.

Take a warm shower or apply warm compresses to trigger letdown.

Massage breasts and then hand express some milk to soften the breast so the infant can "latch on."

Breastfeed long enough to empty breast.

Alternate starting breast.

Take a mild analgesic 20 minutes before feeding if discomfort is pronounced.

Plugged Ducts (Caked Breasts)

Nurse frequently and for long enough to empty the breasts completely.

Rotate feeding position.

Massage breasts prior to feeding, in a warm shower when possible.

Maintain good nutrition and adequate fluid intake.

5. The infant should be burped at regular intervals, preferably at the middle and end of the feeding, or, during the first few feedings, after about every 1/2 oz. If the infant was crying vigorously before feeding, he or she should be burped before feeding or after taking just enough formula to calm down. (See discussion on burping, which follows.)

6. Infants should be encouraged but not forced to feed. Overfeeding can lead to infant obesity.

Burping the Infant

• Burping is done by holding the infant upright on the shoulder or by holding the infant in a sitting position on the feeder's lap with the chin and chest supported by one hand. The back is then stroked or patted gently.

• Newborns frequently regurgitate small amounts. The feeder may find it helpful to keep a "burp cloth" handy. Forceful emesis requires medical evaluation, especially if other symptoms are present.

The Rh-Negative Mother

• A woman who is Rh negative with an indirect Coombs' test negative, and whose infant is Rh positive with a direct Coombs' test negative, is given RhIgG (RhoGAM) within 72 hours after childbirth.

• See Procedure: Administering Rh Immune Globulin (RhIgG, RhoGAM, HypRho-D), on page 282.

Rubella Vaccine

• Women who are not immune to rubella (German measles), as evidenced by a titer of less than 1:10, are usually given the rubella vaccine during the immediate postpartal period because it is known that they are not pregnant.

• Because the rubella vaccine is a live, attenuated vaccine, women are advised not to become pregnant for at least 3 to 4 months after receiving it.

Postpartal Exercises

- The woman should be encouraged to begin simple exercises in the hospital and to continue them at home. Exercise helps to improve muscle tone, contributes to postpartum weight loss, and aids in preventing constipation. Many agencies have a booklet on appropriate exercises.

- Figure 7–3 identifies some commonly used exercises.

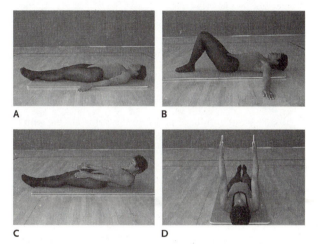

Figure 7–3   Postpartal exercises. Begin with 5 repetitions two or three times daily and gradually increase to 10 repetitions. First day: **A,** Abdominal breathing. Lying supine, inhale deeply using the abdominal muscles. The abdomen should expand. Then exhale slowly through pursed lips, tightening the abdominal muscles. **B,** Pelvic rocking. Lying supine with arms at sides, knees bent, and feet flat, tighten the abdomen and buttocks and attempt to flatten back on floor. Hold for a count of 10, then arch the back, causing the pelvis to "rock." On the second day add: **C,** Chin to chest. Lying supine with legs straight, raise head and attempt to touch chin to chest. Slowly lower head. **D,** Arm raises. Lying supine, arms extended at 90-degree angle from body, raise arms so that they are perpendicular and hands touch. Lower slowly. On fourth day add:

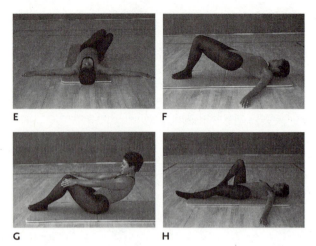

Figure 7–3 (continued) **E,** Knee rolls. Lying supine with knees bent, feet flat, and arms extended to the side, roll knees slowly to one side, keeping shoulders flat. Return to original position and then roll to opposite side. **F,** Buttocks lift. Lying supine, arms at sides, knees bent, and feet flat, slowly raise buttocks and arch the back. Return slowly to the starting position. On the sixth day add: **G,** Abdominal tighteners. Lying supine, knees bent, and feet flat, slowly raise head toward knees. Arms should extend along either side of legs. Return slowly to original position. **H,** Knee to abdomen. Lying supine, arms at sides, bend one knee and thigh until foot touches buttocks. Straighten leg and lower it slowly. Repeat with other leg. After 2 to 3 weeks, more strenuous exercises such as sit-ups and side leg raises may be added as tolerated. Kegel exercises, begun antepartally, should be done many times daily during postpartum to restore vaginal and perineal tone.

Sibling Preparation for the Newborn

- Sibling visits reassure the children that their mother is well and still loves them.

- The parents may ask for advice about dealing with the siblings when mother and baby return from the hospital. The following advice may be helpful:
  1. If possible, have the father carry the new baby inside so that the mother's arms are free to embrace her other children.
  2. Some mothers bring a doll home for the older sibling. The sibling can then care for the doll when the mother is caring for the baby.
  3. Involving older children in baby care helps them develop a sense of closeness with the baby. Even very young children can hold the baby with supervision.
  4. Each parent should spend quality time in a one-to-one experience with each older child. Hugs, kisses, and words of praise are also important.
  5. Regression is common, and a toilet-trained child may regress or may request a bottle for meals.

Care of the Woman Following Cesarean Birth

- The new mother who has given birth by cesarean has postpartal needs similar to those of women who give birth vaginally; however, she also has nursing care needs similar to those of women who have undergone major abdominal surgery.
- Nursing interventions include the following:
  1. Encourage woman to cough, deep breathe, and use incentive spirometry every 2 to 4 hours while awake for the first day or two following birth.
  2. Encourage leg exercises every 2 hours until woman is ambulatory.
  3. Monitor temperature for fever (infection), BP for decrease, and pulse for increase (hemorrhage).
  4. Elevated BP may indicate pregnancy-induced hypertension (PIH) (may occur for up to 48 hours postpartum).

5. Assess for adequate voiding after the Foley catheter is removed. Implement nursing interventions if necessary to encourage voiding (privacy, increased fluid, warm water over perineum, ambulation).

6. Assess for evidence of abdominal distention. *Note* presence or absence of bowel sounds. Measures to prevent or minimize gas pains include leg exercises, abdominal tightening, early ambulation, and avoiding the use of straws.

7. Flatulence may be relieved by lying on the left side, using a rocking chair, and using antiflatulents (such as simethicone), suppositories, and enemas.

8. Encourage shower by second postpartal day (cover incision with plastic wrap until staples are removed and stay close in case woman becomes faint).

9. Measures to alleviate pain include the following:

   a. Administer analgesics as needed. Patient-controlled analgesia (PCA) is frequently used. Epidural morphine may be injected immediately after the cesarean. This method provides pain relief for at least 24 hours.

   b. Offer comfort through positioning, back rubs, oral care, and reduction of noxious stimuli such as noise or odors.

   c. Encourage presence of significant others, including baby.

   d. Encourage breathing, relaxation, and distraction techniques (such as those taught in childbirth preparation classes).

- Provide opportunities for parent-infant interaction.
- Discharge teaching includes need for adequate rest, warning signs of infection, and ways of lifting and feeding infant to avoid strain.

Chapter 8
The At-Risk Postpartal Client

Postpartal Hemorrhage

Overview

The main causes of postpartal hemorrhage are uterine atony (relaxation of uterus due to overdistention of uterus, PIH, intraamniotic infusion, use of magnesium sulfate in labor); retained placental fragments; laceration of genital tract; and vulvar, vaginal, or subperitoneal hematomas and coagulation disorders. Postpartum hemorrhage is characterized by bright-red vaginal bleeding in the presence of either a soft boggy uterus with clots or a well-contracted uterus without clots. This condition most commonly occurs within the first 24 hours after giving birth. Late or delayed hemorrhage occurs after 24 hours after birth, usually within 1 to 2 weeks postpartum, except with subinvolution, when it can occur up to 6 weeks after birth.

Clinical Therapy

1. **Uterine atony.** Oxytocic drugs are administered after separation of the placenta to prevent uterine atony (see Drug Guide: Oxytocin [Pitocin]). Fundal height and firmness are determined; if the uterus is not firm and well contracted after expulsion of the placenta, fundal massage is initiated. If there is excessive bleeding, the clinician may do bimanual uterine compression. Oxygen via mask is administered at 6–10 L/min. Hematocrit, hemoglobin, partial thromboplastin and prothrombin times, and fibrinogen levels are monitored.

Methylergonovine maleate (Methergine) IM (see Drug Guide, on page 275) may be ordered for immediate management of uterine atony.

2. **Retained placental fragments.** Inspect the placenta for any signs that a cotyledon or piece of membrane is missing. If missing pieces are suspected the uterine cavity requires uterine exploration. Sonography may be considered to look for retained fragments. Methylergonovine maleate (Methergine) IM or p.o. (see Drug Guide) is ordered. Prostaglandins (IM or directly injected into the uterine cavity) may be used for rapid sustained contractions.

3. **Lacerations.** Genital tract lacerations should be suspected when vaginal bleeding persists in the presence of a firmly contracted uterus. A visual examination of the cervix is made, and deep cervical lacerations are sutured to stop the bleeding.

4. **Hematomas.** Hematomas present as severe pressure anywhere along the genital tract and purple color to the vaginal mucosa or ecchymotic perineum. Small hematomas are managed with ice packs, analgesia, and ongoing observation. They usually reabsorb naturally. Larger hematomas or those increasing in size are incised, and drained to achieve hemostasis. Bleeding vessels are ligated. Vaginal packing may be inserted to achieve hemostasis if needed. Large vaginal packs can make voiding difficult, and an indwelling catheter is often necessary. Because incision and drainage may predispose the woman to infection, broad-spectrum antibiotics are ordered. Replace blood and clotting factors as needed.

Critical Nursing Assessments

1. Assess BP, pulse, and respirations per postpartum agency protocol. If vaginal bleeding is noted, assess BP, pulse, and respirations every 15 minutes.

2. *Be alert for* hypotension and tachycardia, which can be signs of hypovolemia, along with tachypnea,

decreased BP, pallor, cyanosis, cold and clammy skin, and restlessness.

3. Assess fundal status for height and firmness (see Procedure: Assessing the Fundus Following Vaginal Birth, on page 288). Uterus should be firm and at or below the umbilicus. A well-contracted fundus rules out uterine atony.

4. Assess amount of blood loss/vaginal bleeding and any blood clots expressed.

5. **Assessment technique:** Visual assessment; do pad counts within a given time period or weigh the perineal pads (1 mL of blood weighs 1 g).

6. *Be alert for* blood loss. To determine the amount of blood loss, assess not only the peripads but also the underpads for pooling of blood. To do so, have the woman turn on her side.

7. Examine perineum and buttocks for discoloration, bulging, tender areas. If woman is still recovering from regional anesthesia, frequent visualization of perineum/buttocks is essential. Palpate obvious masses for tenderness and fluctuation.

8. Assess women's pain level. After effects of anesthesia have subsided, vaginal and vulvar hematomas are associated with perineal pain or rectal pressure.

9. Examine vagina or rectum for protruding masses. **Assessment technique:** Position woman on her side, raise her upper buttock, and instruct her to bear down.

10. *Be alert for* bulging purplish mass which may become apparent at the introitus, or a soft mass, which may be palpable upon rectal exam.

11. Assess for bladder distention (hinders effective uterine contractions and involution process).

12. Assess intake and output every 8 hours.

13. *Be alert for* urine output needs to stay at >30 mL/hr to perfuse kidneys well.

14. Assess laboratory results.

15. *Be alert for* decreasing hematocrit (500-mL blood loss may be seen as a 4-point decrease in hematocrit).

16. Assess woman's coping responses, level of understanding of her condition, and emotional status.

17. Assess woman's ability to take care of her baby because of fatigue related to blood loss. Also assess existing support systems at home.

Sample Nursing Diagnoses

- *Fluid volume deficit* related to blood loss secondary to uterine atony, retained placental fragments, lacerations, or hematoma formation.

- *Risk for infection* related to trauma and hemorrhage.

Critical Nursing Interventions

1. Gently massage boggy uterus while supporting lower uterine segment (see Figure 8–1) to stimulate contraction and express clots. *Be alert for* level of massage. Forceful massage can tire the uterus, resulting in uterine atony, and can cause pain. Be gentle. Do not be misled by the fact that a woman has a firm uterus. Significant bleeding can occur from causes other than uterine atony.

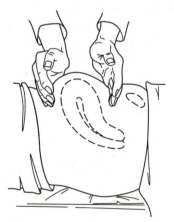

Figure 8–1   Uterine massage

2. Monitor type and amount of bleeding and associated consistency of the uterus. *Be alert for* dark-red blood and relaxed uterus, which indicate uterine atony or retained placental fragments. Bright-red vaginal bleeding and contracted uterus indicate laceration hemorrhage.

3. Apply ice pack during first hour after birth for women at risk for vaginal hematoma. If hematoma forms, use sitz bath after 12 hours.

4. Maintain IV and start second IV with an 18-gauge needle to administer blood products if necessary. Send blood for type and cross match if not already done in the birthing area.

5. Administer oxytocics per order. Carefully note uterine tone and blood pressure response to medication.

6. Monitor intake and output hourly. Initially insert Foley catheter to ensure accurate output determination.

7. Provide oxygen via mask or nasal cannula at 7–10 L/min for signs of respiratory distress.

8. Administer pain medications for discomfort as ordered.

9. Provide stool or chair for use during shower in case of dizziness or weakness to facilitate self-care and progressive ambulation.

10. Review the following critical aspects of the care you have provided:

    • Have I effectively monitored her fundal and lochia status? Did I quickly identify and intervene when there was continued relaxation of the uterus and expression of clots?

    Did I carry out the uterine massage as gently as possible?

    • Are woman's vital signs stable? Is woman showing any signs of hypovolemia?

    • Is woman complaining of discomfort anywhere along the genital tract? Have I provided adequate comfort measures for her, such as cold or warm packs, perineal care, sitz baths, or pain medication?

    • Have I assisted in decreasing the anxiety of the woman and her family by keeping them informed about her status?

- Have I provided the mother with home care information on the following: iron supplementation, expected changes in fundus and lochia, how to massage the fundus as indicated by tone, signs of abnormal bleeding, and when to call health care provider?

Evaluation

- Signs of postpartal hemorrhage are detected quickly and managed effectively.
- Hematoma formation is detected quickly and managed successfully.
- The woman's discomfort is relieved effectively.
- The woman is able to identify abnormal changes that might occur following discharge and understands the importance of notifying her caregiver if they develop.
- Maternal-infant attachment is maintained successfully.

Subinvolution

Overview

Subinvolution is the failure of the uterus to follow the normal pattern of involution and is one of the most common causes of late postpartum hemorrhage. Usually the signs and symptoms of subinvolution are not apparent until about 4 to 6 weeks postpartum. The fundus remains higher in the abdomen/pelvis than expected. Lochia often fails to progress from rubra to serosa to alba. The lochia may remain rubra or return to rubra several days postpartum. Lochia rubra that persists longer than 2 weeks postpartum is highly suggestive of subinvolution. The amount of lochia may be more profuse than expected. Leukorrhea, backache, and foul lochia may occur if infection is present. The woman may also relate a history of irregular or excessive bleeding after the birth.

Clinical Therapy

1. **Uterine examination.** Bimanual uterine exam shows an enlarged, softer than normal uterus.

2. **Drug therapy.** Oral methylergonovine 0.2 mg or ergonovine 0.2 mg q3–4 hrs for 24–48 hours is given to stimulate uterine contractility (see Drug Guide: Methylergonovine Maleate [Methergine] on page 275). Oral antibiotics are ordered if metritis (infection) is present or invasive procedures are done.

3. **Uterine curettage.** If treatment is not effective or if retained placental fragments and polyps are the cause, curettage may be done.

Critical Nursing Assessments

1. Assess characteristics of lochial pattern since birth. *Be alert for* lochia pattern: lochia that does not progress from rubra to serosa or returns to rubra days after the birth.

2. Assess whether mother has felt feverish or has had a temperature. *Be alert for* elevation in temperature, which can occur if infection is the cause of subinvolution.

3. Assess woman's level of understanding regarding her condition, the signs of subinvolution, and when she should call her health care provider.

Sample Nursing Diagnoses

- *Pain* related to stimulation of uterine contraction secondary to administration of oxytocic medications.
- *Risk for infection* related to bacterial invasion of uterus secondary to dilatation and curettage.
- *Health seeking behaviors* related to lack of information about delayed postpartum hemorrhage.

Critical Nursing Interventions

1. During discharge teaching, review normal involution process and progression of lochia from rubra to serosa to alba. Stress that the woman should report any continued bleeding that does not go away with rest and medication and that covers the surface of one perineal pad 2 to 6

weeks after birth. Any adverse effects from the medications should be reported to the health care provider.

2. Discuss the importance of increasing the length and number of rest periods; see if she can have a support person with her during the 24-hour oxytocic medication period. Refer to home care.

3. Inform the lactating woman that she can continue to breastfeed. Low-dose methylergonovine poses no threat to baby, and breastfeeding can assist in involution.

4. If woman has history of elevated blood pressure, teach her the early signs of adverse effects of oxytocic medication on her blood pressure. These signs include nausea, vomiting, headache, and complaints of abdominal cramping or signs of circulatory stasis, including itching, tingling, numbness, and cold fingers and toes.

Sample Nurse's Charting

1930: T 99.2F, P 92, R 16, BP 124/76. Fundus soft 1 FB above symphysis pubis and midline. Tender to palpation. Lochia rubra with small clots. Complains of fatigue, lochia flow return to rubra, and soaking surface of one peripad/day 15 days after birth. Is breastfeeding and expresses concern over continued rubra lochia and progressive fatigue. S. Paulski, RNC

Evaluation

- Woman knows the signs of delayed uterine involution and when to report them to her health care provider.
- Woman understands the treatment regimen and takes her medications as ordered.
- Woman has support to help her deal with increased fatigue and anxiety related to the failure of uterus to return to normal.

Types of Reproductive Tract Infections

Type/Cause	Signs/Symptoms	Treatment
Localized Infection of External Genitals Episiotomy or sutured laceration; infected traumatized perineum, vulva, vagina, or abdominal incision.	Low-grade fever (<38.3°C [101°F]), localized pain, edema, redness, seropurulent discharge. Late: skin discoloration, shock, wound abscess, high temperature, and chills.	Oral antibiotics, removal of stitches to promote drainage, use of saline gauze to keep lesion open, sitz baths, analgesics.
Endometritis (Metritis) Infection of total endrometrium or placental site.	Sawtooth fever pattern (low grade to 103°F [39.4°C]; see Figure 8–2), chills, rapid pulse. Headache, backache, malaise, cramps. Tender uterus. Scant to profuse dark-brown, foul-smelling discharge. In β-hemolytic infection, scant and odorless lochia.	IV antibiotics (cephalosporin or ampicillin), oxytocics to stimulate contraction and lochial drainage, semi-Fowler's position and/or ambulation to promote drainage (aerobic and anaerobic), blood and lochial culture, D&C for retained placental tissue, hydration.
Parametritis (Pelvic Cellulitis) Infection of tissues around uterus via the lymphatics (often following endometritis).	Marked high fever (102–104°F, [38.9–40°C]), chills, abdominal tenderness on one or both sides. Rebound pain during pelvic exam. Vaginal, rectal, abdominal abscesses.	Broad-spectrum antibiotics (IV). Hydration (up to 2000 mL/day), blood transfusion for decreasing hemoglobin, bed rest, analgesics.

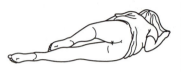

Figure 8–2
Episiotomy is inspected. Woman is on her side, and her upper leg is forward.

Critical Nursing Assessments

1. Assess BP, pulse, and respirations every 2 to 4 hours. Tachycardia is associated with endometritis and pelvic cellulitis.

2. Assess temperature every 4 hours unless elevated, then every 2 hours. **Tip:** Remember that a low-grade fever is common during the first 24 hours after birth. Be alert for elevated temperature (greater than 100.4°F [38°C]) patterns.

3. Assess fundal height, tone, and sensation (see Procedure: Assessing the Fundus Following Vaginal Birth, on page 288). Note any discomfort or pain that is greater than anticipated and note protracted afterpains.

4. Assess perineum every 8 hours. Inspect perineum using good light source. **Assessment technique:** Have woman lie on her side with her top leg slightly forward and ahead of the bottom leg (see Figure 8–2). After donning disposable gloves, lift the buttock to expose the perineum and the anus. If no episiotomy is present the perineum is described as intact. Assess episiotomy or sutured laceration for redness, edema, ecchymosis, discharge, approximation of edges (skin edges together), and tenderness.

5. Assess lochia for type, amount, and odor (see Procedure: Evaluating Lochia after Birth, on page 305).

6. Assess laboratory results for above normal postpartum levels, especially the white blood cell count. **Tip:** Normal postpartum leukocyte levels are already increased (15,000–30,000/mm^3), so be alert for >30,000/mm^3.

7. Assess hydration status.

8. Assess for abscess formation (often a palpable mass and fever).

Sample Nursing Diagnoses

- *Risk for infection* related to broken skin or traumatized tissues.
- *Pain* related to the presence of infection.
- *Altered parenting* related to mother's malaise and other symptoms of infection.

Critical Nursing Interventions

1. Monitor temperature every 4 hours and identify trends. *Be alert for* low-grade fever (<101°F [38.3°C]) with rapid onset, which indicates localized infection. Irregular fever (sawtooth pattern), varying from 101–103°F (38.3–39.4°C) indicates endometritis. Persistent high fever (102–104°F [38.9–40°C]) and chills indicate parametritis.

2. Monitor lochial changes for signs of failure of normal involution.

3. Teach woman about, and perform, proper perineal and hygienic measures to promote healing and prevent contamination of the perineum, such as washing hands frequently and after each peripad change, perineal care (see Chapter 7), and use of sitz baths. Encourage a diet high in protein and vitamin C.

4. Obtain cultures of lochia, wound, and urine (to rule out asymptomatic urinary tract infection). *Tip:* With episiotomy infections, lochia may have a foul odor and appear yellow.

5. Administer antibiotics, oxytocics (see Drug Guide: Oxytocin [Pitocin] and Drug Guide: Methylergonovine Maleate [Methergine]), and analgesic spray as prescribed. Instruct on need to take entire course of prescribed medications at home.

6. Assist mothers with endometritis to ambulate and lie in semi-Fowler's position to facilitate lochial drainage.

7. If parametritis occurs, provide bed rest and maintain IV fluids. Monitor intake and output and urine specific gravity.

8. Teach woman with draining wound or purulent lochia about wound care and proper management of soiled dressings and linen.

9. Institute home care referral as needed.

10. Maintain mother-infant interaction. Assist mother to balance her need for rest and her need for time with her baby.

Evaluation

- The infection is quickly identified and treated successfully without further complications.

- The woman understands the infection and the purpose of therapy; she carries out any ongoing antibiotic therapy if indicated following discharge.

- Maternal-infant attachment is maintained.

Thromboembolic Disease

Overview

Thromboembolic disease refers primarily to superficial thrombophlebitis (thrombus due to inflammation), which primarily forms in saphenous veins, appears on the 3rd or 4th postpartal day, and shows clinical improvement within 48 hours of therapy. Thrombophlebitis often presents as some local heat and redness, mild calf pain, visible and palpable veins, and normal temperature or low-grade fever. Deep vein thrombosis (DVT) is seen in women with a history of thrombosis and increases the likelihood of pulmonary emboli development. Deep vein thrombosis may present with severe leg pain of sudden onset (pain may worsen if leg is in a dependent position and if pressure is applied to calf area), edema and paleness of affected leg, systemic signs of elevated temperature, pulse and chills, and possible positive Homans' signs. Deep vein thrombosis may take up to 4–6 weeks to resolve after the acute symptoms stop.

Clinical Therapy

1. **Superficial thrombophlebitis.** Bed rest with leg elevation is ordered. Moist heat therapy is applied to facilitate

drainage and decrease venous stasis. Elastic support hose are to be worn after acute inflammation subsides.

2. **Deep vein thrombosis.** In addition to treatment for superficial thrombophlebitis, anticoagulant therapy is ordered. Heparin via continuous IV. The desired prothrombin time lab value is 1 1/2–2 1/2 × control in seconds then sodium warfarin (Coumadin) is begun. No aspirin or ibuprofen can be taken by women on anticoagulant therapy. **Special alert:** One percent protamine sulfate is used as the antidote for anticoagulant overdose.

Critical Nursing Assessments

1. Assess vital signs, especially oral temperature, every 4 hours. Be alert for and report temperature > 100.4°F.
2. Assess calves, thighs, and groin area (especially left side) bilaterally for increase in size, color, warmth, peripheral pulses, and positive Homans' sign.

   Assessment technique for Homans' sign: Dorsiflex foot with knee in extended position (see Figure 8–3). If pain occurs in foot or leg with foot dorsiflexion, Homans' sign is positive.
3. Assess CBC, platelet count, and prothrombin time.
4. Assess for evidence of bleeding related to heparin therapy.

Sample Nursing Diagnoses

- *Altered peripheral tissue perfusion* related to obstructed venous stasis.
- *Altered tissue perfusion* related to pulmonary embolism secondary to dislodgement of deep vein thrombus.

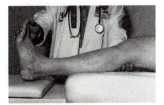

Figure 8–3 Homans' sign: With the woman's knee flexed to decrease the risk of embolization , the nurse dorsiflexes the foot. Pain in the foot or leg is a positive Homans' sign.

Critical Nursing Interventions

1. Monitor vital signs. *Be alert for* elevated temperature, which may be associated with inflammation.

2. Inspect and palpate calf, thigh, and groin area daily for heat, color, tenderness, and peripheral pulses. *Be alert for* increasing redness, swelling, or pain.

3. Monitor any signs of deep vein thrombosis. *Be alert for* sudden onset of severe leg or thigh pain, elevated temperature, or chills. Report these signs to physician immediately.

4. Measure affected portion of leg with nonstretch tape to assess degree of edema.

5. Assist mother to stay on bed rest with her leg fully elevated on pillows. Do not use knee gatch on bed and avoid any pressure on popliteal space (to prevent pelvic pooling and impedance of blood flow). While mother is on bed rest, have her use footboard, do passive exercises, and change position frequently.

6. Apply warm, moist packs to affected leg (vasodilatation facilitates blood flow and decreases pain). Be sure to wrap packs to prevent burns and remove for 10 minutes each hour.

7. Administer antibiotics per order.

8. Administer heparin as ordered after obtaining prothrombin results. Monitor prothrombin and Hct to evaluate bleeding and adequacy of heparinization. Have 1% protamine sulfate on hand for heparin overdose.

9. Initiate progressive ambulation after acute inflammation subsides.

10. Apply support hose (compresses superficial veins and increases deep venous flow).

11. Monitor and report signs of pulmonary emboli. *Be alert for* signs such as vague chest pain, anxiety, respiratory rate >16 breaths/minute, pallor, tachypnea, and possible changes in lung sounds (rales and friction rub).

12. Instruct mother on measures to prevent venous stasis:
    • Avoid crossing legs at the knee while sitting.
    • Elevate the feet while sitting when possible.

- Avoid prolonged standing.
- Ambulate periodically throughout the day.
- Drink at least six 8-oz glasses of water per day.

13. Instruct mother regarding anticoagulant therapy:
    - Take medication at the same time each day.
    - Keep appointments so that clotting times can be monitored and medication can be adjusted.
    - Maintain current eating habits (include green vegetables) and lifestyle.
    - Avoid any activities that may cause bleeding, such as playing contact sports, using stiff toothbrushes, or shaving legs with a straight razor.
    - Be aware of signs of heparin overdose such as bleeding gums, ecchymosis, nosebleed, hematuria, and melena.
    - Note any blood in the stools; it should be reported to the physician.
    - Wear a Medic-Alert bracelet indicating use of anticoagulants.
    - Avoid medications such as aspirin and nonsteriodal antiinflammatory drugs that increase anticoagulant activity.

14. If woman wishes to continue breastfeeding, have her discuss use of low-dose subcutaneous heparin at home rather than warfarin.

15. Review the following critical aspects of the care you have provided:
    - Have I administered the correct dose of heparin at the designated times after first reviewing the results of the clotting studies?
    - Have I been alert for any signs of heparin overdose?
    - What can I do to assist the woman to maintain bed rest?
    - Is the mother able to eat a diet that assists her coagulation status?
    - Have I assessed the woman's understanding of her thrombolic status and answered her questions? Have I given her opportunities to practice preventive measures?

16. Review with the couple the signs and symptoms of thrombophlebitis and the need to report them since the condition may not occur until after discharge. *Tip:* Do not massage affected leg.

Evaluation

- If thrombosis or thrombophlebitis develops, it is detected quickly and managed without further complications.
- At discharge the woman is able to explain the purpose, dosage regimen, and necessary precautions associated with any prescribed medications such as anticoagulants.
- The woman can discuss self-care measures and ongoing therapies (such as the use of elastic stockings) that are indicated.
- The woman has bonded successfully with her newborn and is able to care for the baby effectively.

Urinary Tract Infection

Overview

Most postpartal urinary tract infections (UTIs) are caused by gram-negative organisms such as *Escherichia coli,* which invade the urethra and bladder and cause cystitis. Bladder bacteria then may ascend to the kidney as a result of vesicoureteral reflux during voiding, causing pyelonephritis after several days. Postpartal women are at increased risk because of decreased bladder sensitivity due to stretching, trauma, and retention of residual urine; bacteria introduced during catheterization; and bladder trauma during childbirth. Women may then present with dysuria, urinary urgency and frequency, suprapubic or lower abdominal pain, lower back discomfort, and possibly hematuria. In addition to the signs and symptoms of cystitis, pyelonephritis presents as cloudy urine and systemic signs of high fever, chills, nausea and vomiting (N&V), malaise, fatigue, severe flank pain, and costovertebral angle tenderness (CVAT). Cystitis management must continue after symptoms disappear, since this infection tends to recur.

Clinical Therapy

1. **Urinalysis.** Urinalysis is obtained and analyzed for protein, blood, and organisms. Urine that contains an increase in WBCs ($>100,000$/mL organisms) and protein and/or blood indicates UTI. Urine culture and sensitivities are obtained so organism-specific antibiotics can be identified.

2. **Fluid and drug management.** Fluid intake is increased to 3–4 L/day to dilute the urine and initiate flushing out of the infected urine. Therapeutic doses of vitamin C or cranberry juice are used to acidify the urine. Urine acidification decreases bacterial growth and increases the action of urinary tract antiseptics. Short-acting sulfonamides such as nitrofurantoin (Macrodantin) are ordered except in term pregnancy, when sulfamethoxazole or trimethoprim (Septra, Bactrim) may be given. Urinary tract antiseptics (Azo Gantrisin) or systemic antibiotics (ampicillin or cephalosporins qid for 7–10 days) can also be used. Antispasmotics or urinary analgesics, such as phenazopyridine hydrochloride (Pyridium), may be given to relieve discomfort.

3. **Pyelonephritis management.** If woman develops pyelonephritis, she may be hospitalized for aggressive treatment and monitoring to prevent permanent kidney damage. Intravenous medications are given, and an indwelling bladder catheter may be put in place. Relief of symptoms is usually obtained in 24–48 hours.

Critical Nursing Assessments

1. Assess bladder function for frequency, urgency, and amount of urine output. Inspect urine for color (hematuria), odor, and appearance (concentrated or dilute).

2. Palpate for large mass, at or near umbilicus, that displaces uterine fundus upward, denoting an overdistended bladder.

3. Assess for painful or burning urination.

4. Assess for complaints of suprapubic or lower abdominal discomfort, lower back pain, or severe flank pain.

5. Palpate for costovertebral tenderness.
6. Assess vital signs q4hrs and observe for signs of systemic involvement.
7. Assess intake and output q8hrs.

Sample Nursing Diagnoses

- *Altered urinary elimination* related to urinary tract infection.
- *Risk for injury* related to urinary stasis secondary to overdistention.
- *Health seeking behaviors* related to lack of information about urinary tract infection, its treatment, and its possible sequelae.

Critical Nursing Interventions

1. Obtain clean-catch, midstream sample for urinalysis.
2. Encourage woman to void q2–4hrs and empty bladder completely. Provide ice pack for perineum within 1 hour after birth to decrease edema formation and facilitate voiding.
3. Woman should drink at least eight 10-oz glasses of liquids, especially water, each day. Also encourage woman to drink unsweetened cranberry, plum, apricot, and prune juices, which increase acidity of urine.
4. Provide comfort measures such as back massage and analgesics for back and flank pain, antispasmodics for dysuria and cramping, antiemetics for N&V, and oral hygiene to promote comfort. If woman has a fever provide tepid baths and antipyretics.
5. If woman is taking sulfonamide drugs, instruct her that breastfeeding should be discontinued and teach her how to pump her breasts.

    Be alert for use of sulfonamides. These medications are secreted in breast milk and combine with proteins to create neonatal jaundice; therefore, pumped milk should be discarded while mother is taking these medications.

6. Monitor baby for diarrhea and yeast infections (candidiasis) while mother is taking ampicillin.

7. Instruct mother that her urine may change color with prescribed medication. *Be alert for* the following: Azo Gantrisin can turn urine red or red orange; nitrofurantoin creates brown urine, may cause N&V and diarrhea, and should be taken with food or milk to decrease gastric irritation.

8. Reinforce instruction on prophylactic hygienic practice (eg, wiping from front to back, voiding when she feels the urge to void, wearing cotton underclothing, and voiding after intercourse). Encourage woman to drink two glasses of water immediately after intercourse to increase urine output and flush out contaminants that may have entered the urethra.

Evaluation

- Woman understands any special instructions for taking medications and need for follow-up urine culture.
- Woman knows hygienic, nutritional, and fluid requirements to avoid urinary tract infections and any symptoms to report to health care provider.

Mastitis

Overview

Mastitis refers to an inflammation of the breast commonly caused by *Staphylococcus aureus* and *Haemophilus parainfluenza* from the infant's nose and throat. Contributing factors include clogged milk ducts, lowered maternal defenses due to fatigue or stress, unclean hands, and cracked or fissured nipples. *Candida albicans* is another cause of mastitis. Mastitis usually occurs in the 2nd or 4th week postpartum. A breast abscess may be a complication.

Clinical Therapy

1. **Drug therapy.** Antibiotics are ordered for a full 10-day course even if symptoms subside within a few days.

Antipyretics such as acetaminophen and nonsteriodal antiinflammatory agents are used.

2. **Breastfeeding.** Continued breastfeeding is recommended. In the presence of a yeast infection, the mother and baby are both treated with nystatin for 14 days.

3. **Laboratory tests.** Infectious mastitis is usually indicated by elevated leukocyte and bacterial counts.

4. **Breast abscess management.** If a breast abscess forms, the breast milk and any drainage are cultured. The abscessed area is incised, drained, and packed with sterile gauze.

Critical Nursing Assessments

1. Examine breast for localized redness, tenderness, and swelling. On palpation, it may be very hard and hot, and the lump may feel like a hard moth ball.

2. Inspect nipple for fissures or cracks (entry points for infection). *Be alert for* inflamed and painful nipples, which may indicate a yeast or fungus infection. Breast abscesses appear as hardened, painful local areas of inflammation below the skin surface.

3. Assess mother's general physical status. Systemic symptoms include flulike symptoms: headache, malaise, muscle ache, rapid pulse, and temperature of about 38.5°C (101.3°F).

4. Assess mother's dietary and sleep patterns and level of stress. Decreases in dietary intake and sleep and/or excessive stress and activity can decrease mother's resistance to infection.

5. Assess feeding history for precipitating factors such as ineffective emptying of breasts, engorgement, breast compression from tight clothing or bra, or sudden change in feeding pattern such as baby sleeping through the night or use of supplemental feedings.

6. Inspect baby's mouth for white patches surrounded by redness on the buccal membrane, which indicate presence of *Candida albicans,* or thrush.

Sample Nursing Diagnoses

- *Health seeking behaviors* related to lack of information about appropriate breastfeeding practices.
- *Risk for infection* related to cracked and traumatized breast tissue or nipples.
- *Ineffective breastfeeding* related to pain secondary to development of mastitis.

Critical Nursing Interventions

Preventive Measures

1. Discuss predisposing factors.
2. Use good handwashing technique.
3. Instruct mother about breast care: handwashing before handling breasts or nipples, cleansing of breast with water only (to maintain protective oils), wearing supportive bra at all times (to avoid milk stasis in lower lobes), and changing bra and breast pads frequently.
4. Reinforce mother's knowledge about breastfeeding techniques, such as position, frequency, and removal of baby from breast.
5. Provide special attention to mothers who have blocked milk ducts, which increase the risk for mastitis.

If the Woman has Mastitis

1. Administer oral pain medications as ordered and usually before feeding to ease discomfort.
2. Teach mother to increase feeding frequency, increase fluid intake (six to eight 8-oz glasses a day), have friends or relatives assist with care in order to increase rest periods, breastfeed first on unaffected breast until letdown occurs (promotes complete emptying of both breasts), express milk at least every 3 hours, and massage caked areas toward nipple during feeding (see Figure 8–4).
3. Mother's temperature should be monitored every 4 hours until infection resolves.

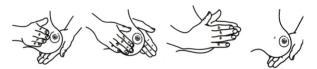

Figure 8–4   Breast massage. Caked areas of breast are massaged toward the nipple.

4. Instruct mother that if there is no improvement within 12–14 hours or if fever persists, she should notify her health care provider. If mother is on antibiotics and the baby develops diarrhea, she should let her physician know.

5. Provide support if mother needs to discontinue breast-feeding temporarily and instruct her on expression of milk.

Evaluation

- The mother is able to identify predisposing factors, signs and symptoms of impending mastitis, and preventive measures.
- Mother knows proper management if mastitis occurs. Mother is supported in her decision to breastfeed and knows how to resume if it is necessary to stop.

Ongoing Management of Selected Perinatal Complications

Pregnancy-Induced Hypertension (PIH)

The postpartum goal is to prevent eclamptic seizures and neurologic sequelae.

Effect of Postpartum on PIH

Postpartum diuresis decreases serum magnesium sulfate levels, thereby increasing the possibility of seizures.

Magnesium sulfate causes uterine relaxation, which increases the possibility of uterine atony; PIH decreases blood volume and lowers platelet counts, which can lead to postpartum hemorrhage.

Critical Nursing Interventions

Monitor vital signs (VS) closely for 48 hours after birth (vital signs should remain stable, then begin to slowly decrease). Monitor urine output (<30 mL/hR) and deep tendon reflexes (DTRs).

Administer IV magnesium sulfate for 24 hours after birth.

Check urine for protein and specific gravity qhR.

Administer diuretic as ordered. Do not give oxytocics because of their hypertensive properties.

Minimize environmental stimuli until status improves.

Have seizure precautions in place.

Monitor for signs of postpartum hemorrhage. Carefully massaging the uterus is important.

Encourage frequent voiding to keep bladder empty and avoid uterine atony.

Emotional support is essential during critical illnesses.

Diabetes

The goal is to maintain normal blood glucose levels, prevent postpartum complications (PIH, hemorrhage, infection), and enhance parent-infant interaction.

Effect of Postpartum on Diabetes

Critical Nursing Interventions

Loss of placental insulin inhibitory hormone (human chorionic somato-mammotrophin [hCS], progesterone) drops insulin requirement sharply. Some women do not require insulin for the first day or so.

Draw blood glucose sample immediately after birth. Monitor urine for glucose and ketones q2hr × 24 hours. Administer insulin on sliding scale based on blood or urine glucose test per physician order.

Increased use of glucose during postpartum.

Monitor for hypoglycemia (see Chapter 2). Maintain IV glucose for 24 hours after birth, then restart diabetic diet.

Increased postpartum complications, such as PIH.

Monitor VS for at least 48 hours. Be alert for PIH symptoms (see Chapter 2).

Hemorrhage due to uterine atony and increased amniotic fluid.

Monitor uterine involution.

Any infection complicates diabetic regulation and increases risk of acidosis.

Maintain excellent handwashing for self. Stress personal hygiene to avoid infections.

Altered parent-infant interaction because baby requires special observation.

Promote flexible visiting policy.

Keep parents informed of baby's progress and status.

If mother is breastfeeding, have her increase her caloric intake by 400–500 kcal/day (20% protein); adjust insulin dosage as needed per physician order. Provide for pumping or breastfeeding opportunities q2–4 hrs around the clock.

Chapter 9

Home Care of the Postpartal Family

Overview

Home care for the postpartal family is focused more on assessment, teaching, and counseling than on physical care. The home setting allows the nurse and family to interact in a more relaxed environment, one in which the family has control. The challenges of assessing and enhancing self-care and/or infant care may be quite unique in the home, and the nurse will have many opportunities to use critical thinking skills to develop creative options with the family.

Planning the Home Visit

The nurse should

- Plan the home visit to occur within 24–48 hours after discharge.
- Make sure the family is consulted regarding a home visit and the time is planned with the family members.
- Explain the purpose of the visit.
- Plan the content to be addressed and gather anticipated materials and equipment.
- Think of ways to create and foster relationships with families.
- Employ safety measures when preplanning and executing the visit.
- Document the visit.
- Provide telephone follow-up.

Maintaining Safety during a Home Visit

Safety is a concern regardless of where nurses are interacting with clients. However, additional precautions can be taken to increase personal safety while out in the community. These precautions include the following:

- Know the specific address and ask a family member for detailed directions to the home.

- Trace the route on a map before leaving and take the map along. Take time to drive around the neighborhood before the visit to identify potential problems.

- Notify someone when you are leaving for a visit and check in with that person as soon as the visit is completed.

- Carry a cellular phone or some method of communication. (Be sure the battery is charged.)

- Lock valuables out of sight in the trunk.

- Carry enough change to make a call from a pay phone if needed.

- Have a working flashlight available, especially if making evening visits.

- Wear a name tag and sensible shoes. Avoid wearing expensive jewelry.

- Be aware of personal body language and alert to the body language of anyone present during the visit, not just the new mother.

- Convey a sense of respect at all times.

- If an occasion occurs that feels unsafe, end the visit.

Nursing Assessments in the Home

- Observe family dynamics. Who is the primary caregiver? Who makes the decisions regarding care of the newborn? Are siblings involved? How are siblings included in interactions and care of the new baby? How is communication shared?

- What information do the parents think they need? It is important to begin with the parents' questions.

Table 9–1   Bath Time Supplies

A plastic tub	Vitamin A and D ointment (for dry skin)
Two bath towels or baby blankets	70% isopropyl alcohol
Two washcloths	Cotton balls or Q-Tips for alcohol application
Mild soap (unperfumed is best because it is not as drying to the baby's skin)	

- Is the home a safe environment for the newborn and the rest of the family? Where does the baby sleep? Are referrals needed and desired?

Home Care of the Newborn

- Review methods of obtaining the newborn's temperature. Provide an opportunity for the parents to demonstrate taking the baby's temperature if they feel comfortable doing so.
- Review holding techniques and determine if the parents have questions.
- Review positioning of the newborn for comfort and safety.
- Review cord care, perineal care with diaper changes, and circumcision care (if applicable).
- Demonstrate a newborn bath if indicated.

Newborn Bath

- Collect supplies (see Table 9–1).
- Advise parents to schedule uninterrupted time for the bath if possible.
- Wash baby's face using a washcloth that has been moistened in warm water but does not contain soap.
- Cleanse eyes first (while the washcloth is the most clean). Using a corner of the washcloth around your finger, wipe

the right eye from the inner canthus to the outer canthus, in one stroke. If another swipe is needed, use another corner of the washcloth. The left eye is washed in the same manner.

- Wash remainder of face, as well as under the chin. Dry. The baby's hair may be washed now or at the end of the bath. (Those most interested in organization and saving steps would say to shampoo the hair now; others would say it needs to be done at the end of the bath to better maintain the newborn's temperature.)

- Wash the chest and abdomen using either lathered hands or a washcloth, then rinse and dry.

- Complete umbilical care by cleansing around the umbilical stump with a cotton ball that has a small amount of alcohol applied.

- Remove diaper. If bathing a male baby, be sure to keep a diaper or rag at hand in case the baby urinates (a male infant is able to spray the urine on a caregiver).

- Gently clean from the area of the symphysis (pubic bone) down toward the anus. Use a separate portion of the washcloth for each motion. The baby's back and buttocks may be washed, rinsed, and dried.

- If the hair has not yet been washed, carefully wrap the baby in a dry blanket. Use a football hold to support the baby safely and yet have one hand free for shampooing. Wet the baby's hair and apply a mild shampoo. Lather, rinse thoroughly, and dry. Brushing the baby's hair stimulates the scalp and also removes dead skin cells and prevents cradle cap.

- Make a hood over the baby's head until he or she is completely dressed and rewarmed after the bath to help retain the infant's body temperature.

- Review procedure for cutting the nails. The nails may be trimmed with special baby-sized cuticle/nail scissors. (Clippers may be too large to allow you to see the baby's nails.)

Home Care of the Mother

- Complete a physical and psychosocial assessment.
- Determine questions the mother has and provide information.
- Reinforce teaching regarding postpartal exercises.
- Discuss infant feeding techniques and provide assistance as needed. See the section on infant feeding in Chapter 7 for additional information.
- Determine if assistance and support for the mother are available and if additional assistance is needed.
- Review signs of illness or problems that need to be referred to the health care provider.
- Talk with the parents to determine if they have questions about resuming sexual activity and if they desire information regarding contraceptive measures.

Resumption of Sexual Activity

- Advise couple to abstain from sexual intercourse until the episiotomy is healed and the lochia has stopped—usually by the end of the 3rd week.
- Some form of water-soluble lubricant such as K-Y jelly may be necessary for intercourse to prevent discomfort because the vagina may be dry (hormone poor).
- Warn breastfeeding couples that the woman may leak milk with orgasm because of the release of oxytocin. Some couples find this pleasurable or amusing; others prefer to have the woman wear a bra. Nursing the baby prior to intercourse may help prevent leaking.
- Point out that the woman may experience decreased interest in sex due to hormonal changes, fatigue, dissatisfaction with her personal appearance, and lingering discomfort (often related to the episiotomy). This may be frustrating, especially for her partner, and the couple may find it helpful to discuss the issue openly.

Table 9–2   Factors to Consider in Choosing a Method of Contraception

Effectiveness of method in preventing pregnancy

Safety of the method:

    Are there inherent risks?

    Does it offer protection against STIs or other conditions?

Client's age and future childbearing plans

Any contraindications in client's health history

Religious or moral factors influencing choice

Personal preferences or biases

Lifestyle:

    How frequently does client have intercourse?

    Does she have multiple partners?

    Does she have ready access to medical care in the event of complications?

    Is cost a factor?

Partner's support and willingness to cooperate

Personal motivation to use method

- To avoid an unplanned pregnancy, advise the couple to use contraception when they resume sexual activity, even if the woman's menses has not yet returned.

Contraception

- Contraceptive information should be made available before the woman is discharged.
- In choosing a method, consistency of use outweighs absolute reliability of a given method.
- Review for the woman (or couple) the advantages and disadvantages of each method, risk factors and contraindications, and the ways of using a given method.
- *Note:* Different methods of contraception may be appropriate at different times in the couple's life. Table 9–2 identifies factors to consider in selecting a method of contraception.

Condom (Male)

- Barrier contraceptive; effectiveness is increased when it is used in combination with a spermicide.
- Advantages:
  1. Small, lightweight, disposable, and inexpensive.
  2. No side effects.
  3. Requires no medical examination or supervision.
  4. Offers visual evidence of effectiveness.
  5. Provides some protection against sexually transmitted infections.
- Disadvantages:
  1. Risk of breakage or displacement.
  2. Possible perineal or vaginal irritation.
  3. Some dulling of sensation.
- Method of use:
  1. Condoms are applied to the erect penis and rolled from the tip to the end of the shaft before vulvar or vaginal contact is made.
  2. A small space is left at the tip to accommodate ejaculate, thereby preventing breakage.
  3. Condom rim should be held when penis is withdrawn from vagina to prevent spillage.
  4. Latex may be weakened by prolonged exposure to heat.
  5. *Note:* Only latex condoms offer protection against HIV/AIDS. "Skin condoms" made of lamb's intestine do not.

Condom (Female)

- Barrier method; not designed to be used with a male condom.
- Advantages:
  1. See male condom.
  2. Because it covers a portion of the woman's perineum and the base of the penis during intercourse, it may

offer increased protection against sexually transmitted infections (STIs).

- Disadvantages:
  1. Higher cost (about $2.25 per condom).
  2. Acceptance by couples not yet established.
- Method of use:
  1. Thin polyurethane sheath with a flexible ring at each end.
  2. Inner ring serves as a means of insertion and covers the cervix like a diaphragm.
  3. Second ring remains outside vagina and covers a portion of the perineum.
  4. Inner sheath prelubricated.
  5. May be inserted up to 8 hours before intercourse (see Figure 9–1).

Diaphragm

- Barrier contraceptive.
- Used with a spermicidal cream or jelly.
- Advantages:
  1. Excellent choice for women who are unable or unwilling to take birth control pills or to have an intrauterine device (IUD).
  2. Involves no medication.
  3. Contraception only used as necessary.
  4. May be inserted up to 4 hours before intercourse.
- Disadvantages:
  1. Women who are not comfortable manipulating their genitals may find it unacceptable.
  2. Some couples feel it interferes with sexual spontaneity.
- Contraindications:
  1. History of toxic shock syndrome.
  2. History of urinary tract infections.
- Method of use:
  1. Must be fitted by a trained caregiver.

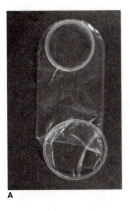

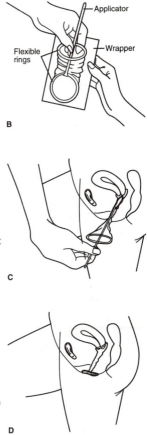

Figure 9–1   A, A female condom. To insert the condom: **B,** Remove the condom and applicator from wrapper by pulling up on ring. **C,** Insert the condom slowly by gently pushing the applicator toward the small of the back. **D,** When the condom is properly inserted, the outer ring should rest on the folds of skin around the vaginal opening, and the inner ring (closed end) should fit loosely against the cervix.

2. Inserted into the vagina prior to intercourse with approximately 1 teaspoonful of spermicidal jelly or cream placed around the rim and in the cup.

3. When correctly placed, it covers the cervix.

4. If more than 4 hours elapse between insertion and intercourse, additional spermicide should be inserted into the vagina (see Figure 9–2).

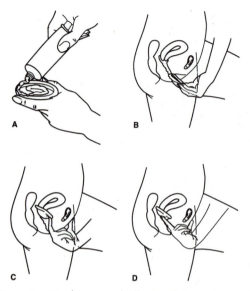

Figure 9–2 Diaphragm and jelly. **A,** Jelly is applied to the rim and center of the diaphragm. **B,** Insertion of the diaphragm. **C,** Rim of the diaphragm is pushed up under the symphysis pubis. **D,** Checking the placement of the diaphragm. Cervix should be felt through the diaphragm.

5. Should be left in place for at least 6–8 hours after intercourse, then removed, cleaned, and allowed to air dry.
6. Must be inspected periodically for holes or tears.

Cervical Cap

- Similar to the diaphragm, except it fits snugly over the cervix.
- May be left in place for up to 48 hours.
- Tends to be more difficult for women to insert and remove.

Fertility Awareness Methods

- Also called natural family planning.
- Advantages:
  1. Free, safe, and acceptable to many whose religious beliefs prohibit other methods.
  2. Involves no artificial substances or medications.
  3. Encourages a couple to communicate about sexual activity and family planning.
  4. Useful in helping a family plan a pregnancy.
- Disadvantages:
  1. Requires extensive initial counseling to use effectively.
  2. May interfere with sexual spontaneity.
  3. Requires extensive maintenance of records for several cycles prior to beginning use.
  4. Difficult for women with irregular cycles to use.
  5. Not as reliable as other methods.
- Method of use: Changes in a woman's cycle (such as changes in mucus, temperature, and other changes) are used to identify fertile and safe days.

Intrauterine Device (IUD)

- Provides continuous contraceptive protection by immobilizing sperm and impeding their progress from the cervix through the uterus to the fallopian tubes.
- May also speed movement of ovum through tubes to uterus.
- Also produces a local inflammatory response.
- Best suited for multiparous women in a monogamous relationship.
- Types available: copper-containing Cu380T (ParaGard), levonorgestrel-releasing intrauterine system (Mirena) and progesterone-containing Progestasert.
- Advantages:
  1. Highly effective.
  2. Continuous contraceptive protection.

   3. No coitus-related activity.
   4. Relatively inexpensive over time.
- Disadvantages:
   1. Increased risk of pelvic inflammatory disease (PID).
   2. Side effects may include severe dysmenorrhea, irregular menses, increased bleeding during menses, uterine perforation, and expulsion.
   3. If IUD fails and pregnancy results, risk of ectopic pregnancy is increased.
- Contraindications:
   1. History of PID.
   2. Not recommended for women with multiple sexual partners because of the increased risk of PID.
- Method of use:
   1. Requires signed consent before insertion by a physician, nurse-midwife, or trained nurse practitioner.
   2. The woman should check for the presence of the string once weekly for the first month and then after each menses.

Oral Contraceptives (OCs) (Birth Control Pills)

- Provide contraceptive protection by inhibiting release of ovum and by maintaining cervical mucus that is hostile to sperm.
- Advantages:
   1. No coitus-related activity.
   2. High effectiveness rate.
   3. Noncontraceptive benefits include decreased menstrual cramps, decreased menstrual flow, increased cycle regularity, decreased incidence of functional ovarian cysts; also substantially reduced incidence of ectopic pregnancy, ovarian cancer, endometrial cancer, iron deficiency anemia, and benign breast disease.
- Disadvantages:
   1. Must be taken daily.

2. Some serious associated side effects, especially those related to thrombus formation.

- Contraindications:
  1. Pregnancy.
  2. Previous history of thrombophlebitis, acute or chronic liver disease, presence of estrogen-dependent carcinoma, undiagnosed uterine bleeding, heavy smoking, hypertension, diabetes, and hyperlipidemia.

- Method of use:
  1. Prescribed after a careful review of the woman's history and a thorough physical exam including blood pressure (BP) check and Pap smear.
  2. Woman seen yearly while on the pill.
  3. Pills are begun on the first Sunday after the beginning of the menstrual cycle and are taken daily for 21 days. The woman then stops for 1 week (or takes seven "blank" pills if she prefers a 28-day package.) She then resumes taking the pills.
  4. Low-dose pills should be taken within 4 hours of the same time daily.
  5. Woman should use a backup method such as condoms during her first cycle on the pills.
  6. If a pill is missed, woman should take it when she remembers and take her pill for the day at the regular time.
  7. Many women take their pills at night, when they are less rushed, and so they are asleep when most side effects (such as nausea) would occur.

Spermicides

- Provide contraceptive protection by destroying sperm or neutralizing vaginal secretions and thereby immobilizing sperm.
- Available in a variety of forms including cream, foam, jelly, film, and suppositories.
- Only minimally effective when used alone. Effectiveness increases when used with a condom.

- Advantages:
  1. Wide availability and low toxicity.
  2. High degree of protection against gonorrhea and some protection against chlamydia, trichomoniasis, and herpes.
- Disadvantages:
  1. Low reliability.
  2. Some messiness.

Long-Acting Progestin Contraceptives

- Types:
  1. Subdermal implants (Norplant). Six silastic capsules of levonorgestrel, a progestin, are implanted in the woman's arm. Effective for up to 5 years. Requires a minor surgical procedure for insertion.
  2. Depot-medroxyprogesterone acetate (DMPA) (Depo-Provera). Given as a singular IM injection every 3 months.
- Method of action:
  1. Prevents ovulation in most women.
  2. Also stimulates the production of thick cervical mucus, which inhibits sperm penetration.
- Advantages:
  1. Provides continuous contraception that is removed from the act of coitus.
  2. Long acting.
- Disadvantages:
  1. Variety of side effects (spotting or irregular bleeding, amenorrhea, weight gain, increased incidence of ovarian cysts, hirsutism, headaches, depression).
  2. Implants may be visible in very slender users; may be difficult to remove.
  3. With DMPA return of fertility may be delayed up to 5 months.

Lunelle (Medroxyprogesterone Acetate and Estradiol Cypionate)

- Approved by FDA in 2000.
- Highly effective monthly IM injection.
- Side effect pattern similar to that of OCs.

Vasectomy

- Male sterilization procedure in which the vas deferens is severed surgically.
- Relatively simple procedure that does not interfere with erectile function.
- Should be considered irreversible, despite some success with microsurgical techniques to reverse the operation.

Tubal Ligation

- Female sterilization procedure in which the fallopian tubes are severed.
- Because it involves general anesthesia, it has more associated risks than vasectomy.
- Should be considered irreversible, despite some success with microsurgical techniques to reverse the operation.

Betamethasone (Celestone Solupan)

Pregnancy Risk Category: C

Overview of Maternal-Fetal Action

Studies have provided ample evidence that glucocorticoids such as betamethasone are capable of inducing pulmonary maturation and decreasing the incidence of respiratory distress syndrome in preterm infants. The mechanism by which corticosteroids accelerate fetal lung maturity is unclear, but it is related to the stimulation of enzyme activity by the drug. The enzyme is required for biosynthesis of surfactant by the type II pneumocytes. Surfactant is essential to the proper functioning of the lung in that it decreases the surface tension of the alveoli. Glucocorticoids also increase the rate of glycogen depletion, which leads to thinning of the interalveolar septa and increases the size of the alveoli. The thinning of the epithelium brings the capillaries into closer proximity with the air spaces and improves oxygen exchange.

Route, Dosage, Frequency

Prenatal maternal intramuscular injections of 12 mg of betamethasone are given once a day for 2 days. Dexamethasone may also be given in doses of 6 mg every 6 hours for four doses (Guinn & Lee, 2000). To obtain maximum results, birth should be delayed for at least 24 hours after completing the first round of treatment. The effect of corticosteroids may be transient. Currently, it is suggested by some that the treatment regimen be repeated every week up to 34 weeks' gestation for the undelivered fetus with an immature lung profile, but this approach is controversial (Guinn & Lee, 2000).

Contraindications

Inability to delay birth

Adequate L/S ratio

Presence of a condition that necessitates immediate birth (eg, maternal bleeding)

Presence of maternal infection, diabetes mellitus, hypertension

Gestational age greater than 34 completed weeks

Maternal Side Effects

Increased risk for infection has not been supported in large studies. There may, however, be some increase in the incidence of infection in women with premature rupture of the membranes. Maternal hyperglycemia may occur during corticosteroid administration. Insulin-dependent diabetics may require insulin infusions for several days to prevent ketoacidosis. Corticosteroids may increase the risk of pulmonary edema, especially when used concurrently with tocolytics (Iams, 1996a; National Institute of Health, 1994).

Effects on Fetus or Neonate

Lowered cortisol levels at birth, but rebound occurs by 2 hours of age

Hypoglycemia

Increased risk of neonatal sepsis

Animal studies have shown serious fetal side effects such as reduced head circumference, reduced weight of the fetal adrenal and thymus glands, and decreased placental weight. Human studies have not shown these effects, however.

Nursing Considerations

Assess for presence of contraindications.

Provide education regarding possible side effects.

Administer betamethasone deep into gluteal muscle, avoiding injection into deltoid (high incidence of local atrophy). (Dexamethasone may be administered IM or IV.)

Periodically evaluate BP, pulse, weight, and edema.

Assess lab data for electrolytes and blood glucose level.

Although concomitant use of betamethasone and tocolytic agents has been implicated in increased risk of pulmonary edema, the betamethasone has little mineral corticoid activity; therefore, it probably does not add significantly to the salt and water retention effects of β-adrenergic agonists. Other causes of noncardiogenic pulmonary edema should also be investigated if pulmonary edema develops during administration of betamethasone to a woman in preterm labor.

Dinoprostone (Cervidil) Vaginal Insert

Pregnancy Risk Category: C

Overview of Maternal-Fetal Action

Dinoprostone is a naturally occurring form of prostaglandin E_2. Dinoprostone can be used at term to ripen the cervix and can stimulate the smooth muscle of the uterus to enhance uterine contractions. A single vaginal insert may be used to ripen the cervix, and then oxytocin can be administered. (Forrest Pharmaceuticals, Inc. Drug Insert, 1995; Zatuchi & Slupik, 1996).

Route, Dosage, Frequency

The vaginal insert contains 10 mg of dinoprostone. The insert is placed transversely in the posterior fornix of the vagina, and the client is kept supine for 2 hours but then may ambulate. The dinoprostone is released at approximately 0.3 mg/hr over a 12-hour period. The vaginal insert should be removed by pulling on the retrieval string upon onset of uterine contractions or after 12 hours (Forrest Pharmaceuticals, Inc. Drug Insert, 1995).

Contraindications

- Client with known sensitivity to prostaglandins
- Presence of fetal distress
- Unexplained bleeding during pregnancy
- Strong suspicion of cephalopelvic disproportion
- Client already receiving oxytocin
- Client with six or more previous term pregnancies
- Client who is not anticipated to be able to give birth vaginally

Dinoprostone vaginal insert should be used with *caution* in clients with ruptured membranes, a fetus in breech presentation, presence of glaucoma, or history of asthma (Forrest Pharmaceuticals, Inc. Drug Insert, 1995).

Maternal Side Effects

Uterine hyperstimulation with or without fetal distress has occurred in a very small number (2.8%–4.7%) of clients. Fewer than 1% of clients have experienced fever, nausea, vomiting, diarrhea, or abdominal pain (Forrest Pharmaceuticals, Inc. Drug Insert, 1995).

Effects on Fetus or Neonate

Fetal distress (Zatuchi & Slupik, 1996).

Nursing Considerations

- Assess for presence of contraindications.
- Monitor maternal vital signs, cervical dilatation, and effacement carefully.
- Monitor fetal status for presence of reassuring fetal heart rate pattern (baseline 120–160 bpm presence of short-term variability, average variability, presence of accelerations with fetal movement, absence of late or variable decelerations).
- Remove vaginal insert if uterine hyperstimulation, sustained uterine contractions, fetal distress, or any other maternal adverse actions occur.

Erythromycin Ophthalmic Ointment (ILotycin Ophthalmic)

Overview of Neonatal Action

Erythromycin (llotycin Ophthalmic) is used as prophylactic treatment of ophthalmia neonatorum, which is caused by the bacteria *Neisseria gonorrhoeae.* Preventive treatment of gonorrhea in the newborn is required by law. Erythromycin is also effective treatment against ophthalmic chlamydial infections. It is either bacteriostatic or bactericidal, depending on the organisms involved and the concentration of drug.

Pregnancy risk category: C

Route, Dosage, Frequency

Ophthalmic ointment (0.5%) is instilled as a narrow ribbon or strand, 1/4 in long, along the lower conjunctival surface of each eye, starting at the inner canthus. It is instilled only once in each eye. The ointment may be administered in the birthing area or, alternatively, later in the nursery so that eye contact between infant and parent is facilitated and the bonding process immediately after birth is not interrupted.

Neonatal Side Effects

Sensitivity reaction; such as edema, inflammation, or drainage may interfere with ability to focus and may cause edema and inflammation. Side effects usually disappear in 24 to 48 hours.

Nursing Considerations

- Wash hands immediately prior to instillation to prevent introduction of bacteria.
- Clean the newborn's eyes to remove any drainage.
- Use new tube or single-use container for ophthalmic ointment administration shortly after birth.
- Massage eyelids gently to distribute the ointment (Zenk, Sills, & Koeppel, 1999).
- May wipe away excess after 1 minute (AAP, 1997).
- Do not irrigate the eyes after instillation.
- Observe for hypersensitivity.
- Teach parents about need for eye prophylaxis. Educate them regarding side effects and signs that need to be reported to the health care provider.

Magnesium Sulfate (MgSO$_4$)

Pregnancy Risk Category: B

Overview of Obstetric Action

MgSO$_4$ acts as a central nervous system (CNS) depressant by decreasing the quantity of acetylcholine released by motor nerve impulses and thereby blocking neuromuscular transmission. This action reduces the possibility of convulsion, which is why MgSO$_4$ is used in the treatment of preeclampsia. Because magnesium sulfate secondarily relaxes smooth muscle, it may decrease the blood pressure, although it is not considered an antihypertensive. MgSO$_4$ may also decrease the frequency and intensity of uterine contractions; as a result it is also used as a tocolytic in the treatment of preterm labor.

Route, Dosage, Frequency

MgSO$_4$ is generally given intravenously to control dosage more accurately and prevent overdosage. An occasional physician still prescribes intramuscular administration. However, it is painful and irritating to the tissues and does not permit the close control that intravenous (IV) administration does. The intravenous route allows for immediate onset of action. It must be given by infusion pump for accurate dosage.

For Treatment of Preterm Labor

Loading dose: 4–6 g MgSO$_4$ in 250 mL solution administered over a 20-minute period.

Maintenance dose: 1–4 g/hr via infusion pump (Creasy & Iams, 1999).

For Treatment of Preeclampsia

Loading dose: 2–4 g MgSO$_4$ is administered over a 5-minute period.

Maintenance dose: 1 g/hr via infusion pump (Roberts, 1999).

Note: MgSO$_4$ is excreted via the kidneys. Because women in preterm labor typically have normal renal function, they generally require higher levels of magnesium to achieve a therapeutic range than women who have preeclampsia and may have compromised renal function. Maintenance dose may need to be adjusted based on serum magnesium levels.

Maternal Contraindications

Diagnosed maternal myasthenia gravis is the only absolute contraindication to the administration of $MgSO_4$. A history of myocardial damage or heart block is a relative contraindication to use of the drug because of the effects on nerve transmission and muscle contractility. Extreme care is necessary in administration to women with impaired renal function because the drug is eliminated by the kidneys, and toxic magnesium levels may develop quickly.

Maternal Side Effects

Most maternal side effects are dose related. Lethargy and weakness related to neuromuscular blockade are common. Sweating, a feeling of warmth, flushing, and nasal congestion may be related to peripheral vasodilation. Other common side effects include nausea and vomiting, constipation, visual blurring, headache, and slurred speech. Signs of developing toxicity include depression or absence of reflexes, oliguria, confusion, respiratory depression, circulatory collapse, and respiratory paralysis. Rapid administration of large doses may cause cardiac arrest.

Effects on Fetus or Neonate

The drug readily crosses the placenta. Some authorities suggest that transient decrease in fetal heart rate (FHR) variability may occur; others report that no change occurred. In general $MgSO_4$ therapy does not pose a risk to the fetus. Occasionally, the newborn may demonstrate neurologic depression or respiratory depression, loss of reflexes, and muscle weakness. Ill effects in the newborn may actually be related to fetal growth retardation, prematurity, or perinatal asphyxia.

Nursing Considerations

1. Monitor the blood pressure closely during administration.
2. Monitor maternal serum magnesium levels as ordered (usually every 6–8 hours). Therapeutic levels are in the range of 4.8–9.6 mg/dL. Reflexes often disappear at serum magnesium levels of 8–12 mg/dL; respiratory depression occurs

at levels of 15–17 mg/dL; cardiac arrest occurs at levels above 30 mg/dL (Sibai, 1996; Silver, 1996).

3. Monitor respirations closely. If the rate is less than 12/minute, magnesium toxicity may be developing, and further assessments are indicated. Many protocols require stopping the medication if the respiratory rate falls below 12/minute.

4. Assess knee jerk (patellar tendon reflex) for evidence of diminished or absent reflexes. Loss of reflexes is often the first sign of developing toxicity. Also note marked lethargy or decreased level of consciousness and hypotension.

5. Determine urinary output. Output less than 30 mL/hr may result in the accumulation of toxic levels of magnesium.

6. If the respirations or urinary output fall below specified levels or if the reflexes are diminished or absent, no further magnesium should be administered until these factors return to normal.

7. The antagonist of magnesium sulfate is calcium. Consequently, an ampule of calcium gluconate should be available at the bedside. The usual dose is 1 g given IV over a period of about 3 minutes.

8. Monitor fetal heart tones continuously with IV administration.

9. Continue $MgSO_4$ infusion for approximately 24 hours after birth as prophylaxis against postpartum seizures if given for pregnancy-induced hypertension (PIH).

10. If the mother has received $MgSO_4$ close to birth, the newborn should be closely observed for signs of magnesium toxicity for 24–48 hours.

Note: Protocols for magnesium sulfate administration may vary somewhat according to agency policy. Consequently, individuals are referred to their own agency protocols for specific guidelines.

Methylergonovine Maleate (Methergine)

Overview of Action

Methylergonovine maleate (Methergine) is an ergot alkaloid that stimulates smooth muscle tissue. Because the uterus is especially sensitive to this drug, it is used postpartally to stimulate the uterus to contract in order to decrease blood loss by clamping off uterine blood vessels and to promote involution. In addition, the drug has a vasoconstrictive effect on all blood vessels, especially the larger arteries. This may result in hypertension, particularly in a woman whose blood pressure is already elevated.

Route, Dosage, Frequency

Methergine has a rapid onset of action and may be given orally or intramuscularly.

Usual IM dose: 0.2 mg following delivery of the placenta. The dose may be repeated every 2–4 hours if necessary.

Usual oral dose: 0.2 mg every 4 hours (six doses).

Maternal Contraindications

Pregnancy, hepatic or renal disease, cardiac disease, and hypertension or pregnancy-induced hypertension contraindicate use of this drug. Methylergonovine maleate must be used with caution during lactation (Karch, 2001).

Maternal Side Effects

Hypertension, nausea, vomiting, headache, bradycardia, dizziness, tinnitus, abdominal cramps, palpitations, dyspnea, chest pain, and allergic reactions may be noted.

Effects on Fetus or Neonate

Because Methergine has a long duration (3 hours [Karch, 2000]) and action and can thus produce tetanic contractions, it **should never be used during pregnancy or in labor,** when it may result in a sustained uterine contraction that may cause amniotic fluid embolism (increased pressure in uterus may allow entry of amniotic fluid under the edge of the placenta and thus entry into the maternal venous system), uterine rupture, cervical and perineal lacerations (resulting from tetanic contractions and rapid birth of the baby), and hypoxia and intracranial hemorrhage in the baby (because of tetanic contractions, which severely decrease the maternal-placental-fetal blood flow, or uterine rupture, which causes cessation of blood flow to the unborn baby) (PDR Nurse's Handbook, 2001).

Nursing Considerations

- Monitor fundal height and consistency and the amount and character of the lochia.
- Assess the blood pressure before and routinely throughout drug administration.
- Observe for adverse effects or symptoms of ergot toxicity (ergotism) such as nausea and vomiting, headache, muscle pain, cold or numb fingers and toes, chest pain, and general weakness (PDR Nurse's Handbook, 2001).
- Provide client and family teaching regarding importance of not smoking during Methergine administration (nicotine from cigarettes leads to constricted vessels and may lead to hypertension), signs of toxicity.

Naloxone Hydrochloride (Narcan)

Overview of Neonatal Action

Naloxone hydrochloride (Narcan) is used to reverse respiratory depression due to acute narcotic toxicity. It displaces morphine-like drugs from receptor sites on the neurons; therefore the narcotics can no longer exert their depressive effects. Naloxone reverses narcotic-induced respiratory depression, analgesia, sedation, hypotension, and pupillary constriction.

Route, Dosage, Frequency

Intravenous dose is 0.1 to 0.2 mg/kg (0.25 to 0.5 mL/kg of 0.4 mg/mL preparation) concentration at birth, including premature infants. This drug is usually given through the umbilical vein or endotracheal tube, although naloxone can be given intramuscularly or subcutaneously. The use of "neonatal" naloxone (Narcan 0.02 mg/mL) is discouraged because of the extremely large fluid volumes that are needed.

Reversal of drug depression occurs within 1–2 minutes after IV administration. The duration of action is variable (minutes to hours) and depends on the amount of the drug present and the rate of excretion. Dose may be repeated in 3–5 minutes. If there is no improvement after two or three doses, discontinue naloxone administration. If initial reversal occurs, repeat dose as needed.

Neonatal Contraindications

Naloxone should not be administered to infants of narcotic-addicted mothers because it may precipitate acute withdrawal syndrome (increased HR and BP, vomiting, tremors).

Respiratory depression may result from nonmorphine drugs, such as sedatives, hypnotics, anesthetics, or other nonnarcotic CNS depressants.

Neonatal Side Effects

Excessive doses may result in irritability, increased crying, and possible prolongation of partial thromboplastin time (PTT).

Tachycardia may occur.

Nursing Considerations

- Monitor respirations closely—rate and depth.
- Assess for return of respiratory depression when naloxone effects wear off and effects of longer-acting narcotics reappear.
- Have resuscitative equipment, O_2, and ventilatory equipment available.
- Monitor bleeding studies.
- Note that naloxone is incompatible with alkaline solutions.
- Store at room temperature and protect from light.
- Compatible with heparin.

Postbirth Epidural Morphine

Overview of Action

Epidural morphine is used to provide relief of pain associated with cesarean birth, extensive episiotomies (mediolaterals), or third- and fourth-degree lacerations. Epidural morphine pain relief results directly from its effect on the opiate receptors in the spinal cord (it depresses pain impulse transmission). Morphine binds opiate receptors, thereby altering both the perception of and the emotional response to pain. Women experience little or no discomfort or pain during recovery and for up to 24 hours afterward. There is no motor or sympathetic block or associated hypotension. Onset of analgesia is slower, but duration is longer.

Dosage, Route

5–10 mg of morphine is injected through a catheter into the epidural space, providing relief for about 24 hours (Wilson, Shannon, & Strang, 2001).

Maternal Contraindications

Hypersensitivity to opiates

Narcotic addiction

Chronic debilitating respiratory disease

Reduced blood volume

Maternal Side Effects

Late-onset respiratory depression (rare but may occur 8–12 hours after administration)

Nausea and vomiting (occurring between 4 and 7 hours after injection)

Itching (begins within 3 hours and lasts up to 10 hours)

Urinary retention

Somnolence (rarely)

Side effects can be managed with naloxone (Cunningham et al., 1997)

Effect on Fetus or Neonate

No adverse effects since medication is injected after birth of baby

Nursing Considerations

Assess client's sensitivity to narcotics on admission.

Monitor and evaluate analgesic effect. Ask client about comfort level and notify anesthesiologist of inadequate pain relief.

If present, check epidural catheter for obvious knots, breaks, and leakage at insertion site and catheter hub.

Assess for pruritus (scratching and rubbing, especially around the face and neck).

Administer comfort measures for narcotic-induced pruritus, such as lotion, back rubs, cool or warm packs, or diversional activities. If the itching can be tolerated, naloxone should be avoided, especially because it counteracts the pain relief.

If allergic reaction (urticaria, edema, or respiratory difficulties) occurs, administer naloxone or diphenhydramine per physician order.

Provide comfort measures for nausea or vomiting, such as frequent oral hygiene or gradual increase in activity; administration of naloxone, trimethobenzamide, or metoclopramide HCI per physician order.

Assess postural blood pressure and heart rate before ambulation.

Assist client with her first ambulation and then as needed.

Assess respiratory function frequently for the first 24 hours, then every 2–8 hours as needed. Also assess level of consciousness and mucous membrane color. May need to monitor client via apnea monitor for 24 hours and use continuous pulse oximetry.

Monitor urinary output and assess bladder for distension. Assist client to void.

Vitamin K₁ Phytonadione (AquaMEPHYTON)

Overview of Neonatal Action

Phytonadione is used in prophylaxis and treatment of hemorrhagic disease of the newborn. It promotes liver formation of the clotting factors, II, VII, IX, and X. At birth, the neonate does not have the bacteria in the colon that are necessary for synthesizing fat-soluble vitamin K_1, therefore, the newborn may have decreased levels of prothrombin during the first 5 to 8 days of life, reflected by a prolongation of prothrombin time.

Route, Dosage, Frequency

Intramuscular injection is given in the vastus lateralis thigh muscle. A one-time-only prophylactic dose of 0.5 to 1 mg is given in-

tramuscularly in the birthing area or within 1 hour of birth
(Zenk, Sills, & Koeppel, 1999).

If the mother received anticoagulants during pregnancy, an additional dose may be ordered by the physician and is given at
6 to 8 hours after the first injection. IM/SC concentration:
1 mg/0.5 mL (neonatal strength); can use 10 mg/mL concentration to minimize volume injected.

Neonatal Side Effects

Pain and edema may occur at injection site. Allergic reactions,
such as rash and urticaria, may also occur.

Nursing Considerations

- Protect drug from light.
- Give vitamin K_1 before circumcision procedure.
- Observe for signs of local inflammation.
- Observe for jaundice and severe hemolytic anemia, especially
  in preterm infants.
- Observe for bleeding (usually occurs on second or third day).
  Bleeding may be seen as generalized ecchymoses or bleeding
  from umbilical cord, circumcision site, nose, or gastrointesti-
  nal tract. Results of serial PT and PTT should be assessed.

Administration of Rh Immune Globulin (RhIgG) (RhoGAM, HypRho-D)

Nursing Action

Objective: Confirm that Rh immune globulin is indicated.

Confirm that mother is Rh negative by checking her prenatal or intrapartal record. Then confirm that sensitization has not occurred—maternal indirect Coombs' negative.

Confirm that infant is Rh positive. (A sample of the infant's cord blood is generally sent to the lab immediately after birth for typing and cross matching.) If infant is Rh positive, confirm that sensitization has not occurred—direct Coombs' negative.

Objective: Confirm that the woman does not have a history of allergy to immune globulin preparations.

Review entries on medication allergies in client chart and ask woman specifically whether she has had any allergic reactions to medications, globulins, or blood products.

Rationale

Sensitization occurs when an Rh-negative woman is exposed to Rh-positive blood. She develops antibodies to the Rh-positive blood. These antibodies can attack the fetal red blood cells, causing profound anemia. If both the direct and indirect Coombs' tests are negative, sensitization has not occurred, and Rh immune globulin is indicated.

Rh immune globulin is made from the plasma portion of blood. Allergic reactions are possible.

Objective: Explain purpose and procedure. Have consent signed.

The woman should clearly understand the purpose of the procedure, its rationale, and the procedure itself, including any risks. Generally, the primary side effects are erythema and tenderness at the injection site and allergic responses.

Many agencies require informed consent before administering Rh immune globulin.

Objective: Obtain correct medication.

Because blood products are involved in the preparation, careful verification is essential.

Rh immune globulin is available from the blood bank or pharmacy according to agency policy. Lot numbers for the drug and the cross match should be the same.

Objective: Confirm client identity and administer medication in deltoid muscle.

The medication causes passive immunity to occur and "tricks" the body into believing that it is not necessary to develop antibodies. Immunization is indicated any time there is a potential for maternal exposure to Rh-positive blood. It is given prophylactically at 28 weeks' gestation, within 72 hours after the birth of an Rh-positive Coombs' negative child, and following any spontaneous or therapeutic abortion, ectopic pregnancy, or amniocentesis.

Medication is administered intramuscularly within 72 hours of childbirth. The normal dose of 300 µg provides passive immunity following exposure of up to 15 mL of transfused RBCs or 30 mL of fetal blood. If a larger bleed is suspected (as in cases of severe abruptio placentae), additional doses may be administered at one time using multiple sites or at regular intervals as long as all doses are given within 72 hours of childbirth.

(continued)

Administration of Rh Immune Globulin (continued)

Nursing Action	Rationale
Objective: Complete education for self-care.	
Provide opportunities for the woman to ask questions and express concerns.	Many women, especially primigravidas, are not aware of the risks for an Rh-positive fetus of a sensitized Rh-negative mother. They must understand the importance of receiving medication for each pregnancy to ensure continued protection.
Objective: Complete client record.	
Chart according to agency procedure. Most agencies chart lot number, route, dose, client education.	Provides a permanent record.

Assessing Deep Tendon Reflexes and Clonus

Nursing Action

Objective: Assemble and prepare equipment.

Obtain a percussion hammer. If one is not available, the side of the hand is also useful in assessing deep tendon reflexes (DTRs).

Objective: Prepare woman.

Explain the procedure, indications for it, and information that will be obtained. At a minimum, check the patellar reflex. Most nurses check a second reflex, such as the biceps, triceps, or brachioradialis.

Objective: Elicit reflexes.

Patellar reflex. The woman is positioned with her legs hanging over the edge of the bed (feet should not be touching the floor). She may also lie supine with her knees slightly flexed and supported by the nurse. The nurse briskly strikes the

Rationale

A percussion hammer permits accurate delivery of a brisk tap.

Explanation decreases anxiety and increases cooperation. DTRs are assessed to gain information about CNS status and to assess the effects of $MgSO_4$ if the woman is receiving it.

Correct positioning and technique are essential to elicit the reflex. The correct position causes the muscle to be slightly stretched. Then when the tendon is stretched with the tap, the muscle should contract.

(continued)

Assessing Deep Tendon Reflexes and Clonus (continued)

Nursing Action

patellar tendon, which is located just below the patella. Normal response is extension or a thrusting forward of the foot.

Biceps reflex. The woman's arm is flexed at the elbow with the nurse's thumb placed on the biceps tendon. The nurse's thumb is struck in a slightly downward motion and response is assessed. Normal response is flexion of the arm.

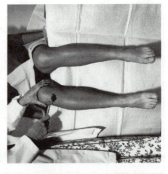

Correct sitting position for eliciting patellar reflex.

Objective: Grade reflexes.

Reflexes are graded on a scale of 0 to 4+. See Table 13–2 on page 314 of textbook.

Normally reflexes are 1+ or 2+. With CNS irritation, hyperreflexia may be present; with high magnesium levels, reflexes may be diminished or absent.

Objective: Assess for clonus.

With the knee flexed and the leg supported, vigorously dorsiflex the foot, maintain the dorsiflexion momentarily, and then release.

Clonus indicates more pronounced hyperreflexia and is indicative of CNS irritability.

Normal response: The foot returns to its normal position of plantar flexion. Clonus is present if the foot "jerks" or taps against the examiner's hand. If so, the number of taps or beats of clonus is recorded.

To elicit clonus, sharply dorsiflex the foot.

Objective: Report and record findings.

For example: DTRs 2+, no clonus or DTRs 4+, 2 beats clonus.

Provides a permanent record.

Assessing the Fundus Following Vaginal Birth

Nursing Action

Objective: Prepare the woman.

- Explain the procedure.
- Ask the woman to void.
- Position the woman flat in bed with her head comfortably on a pillow. If the procedure is uncomfortable, the woman may flex her legs.

Objective: Determine uterine firmness.

- Gently place one hand on the lower segment of the uterus. Using the side of the other hand, palpate the abdomen until you locate the top of the fundus.
- Determine whether the fundus is firm. If it is not firm, massage the abdomen lightly until the fundus is firm.

Objective: Determine the height of the fundus.

Measure the top of the fundus in finger breadths above, below, or at the umbilicus.

Rationale

Explanation decreases anxiety and increases cooperation.
A full bladder will cause uterine atony.
The supine position prevents falsely high assessment of fundal height.
Flexing the legs relaxes the abdominal muscles.

This position provides support for the uterus and a larger surface for palpation.

A firm fundus indicates that the muscles are contracted and bleeding will not occur.

Fundal height gives information about the progress of involution.

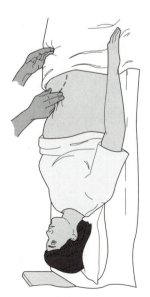

Measurement of descent of fundus for the woman with vaginal birth. The fundus is located two finger breadths below the umbilicus.

Objective: Ascertain the position of the fundus.

- Determine whether the fundus has deviated from the midline. If it is not in the midline, locate the position. Evaluate the bladder for distention.

- Measure urine output for the next few hours until normal elimination status is established.

The fundus may be deviated when the bladder is full.

(continued)

Assessing the Fundus Following Vaginal Birth (continued)

Nursing Action	Rationale
Objective: Correlate the uterine status with lochia.	
Observe the amount, color, and odor of the lochia and the presence of clots.	As normal involution occurs, the lochia decreases and changes from rubra to serosa. Increased amounts of lochia may be associated with uterine relaxation; failure to progress to the next type of lochia may indicate uterine relaxation or infection.
Objective: Record the findings.	
• Fundal height is recorded in finger breadths (e.g., "2 FB ↓ U; 1 FB ↑ U").	Provides a permanent record.
• If massage was necessary: "Uterus: Boggy → firm c̄ light massage."	

Assisting during Amniocentesis

Nursing Action

Objective: Prepare the woman.

- Explain the procedure and reassure the woman.
- Ask the woman to sign a consent form.

Objective: Assemble the equipment.

Prepare and arrange the following items so they are easily accessible:

- 22-gauge spinal needle with stylet
- 10 and 20-mL syringes
- 1% xylocaine
- Povidone-iodine (Betadine)
- Three 10-mL test tubes with tops (amber colored or covered with tape)

Objective: Monitor the woman's vital signs.

Obtain baseline data on maternal BP, temperature, pulse, respirations, and FHR; then monitor every 15 minutes.

Rationale

Explanation of the procedure decreases anxiety.

It is the physician's responsibility to obtain informed consent. The woman's signature indicates her awareness of risks and gives her consent to the procedure.

Amniotic fluid must be shielded from light to prevent breakdown of bilirubin.

(continued)

Assisting during Amniocentesis (continued)

Nursing Action

Objective: Locate the fetus and the placenta.

Assist with real-time ultrasound to assess needle insertion during the procedure.

Objective: Cleanse the woman's abdomen.

Objective: Collect the amniotic fluid specimen.

- Obtain the test tubes from the physician.
- Label the tubes with the correct identification and send to the lab with the appropriate lab slips.

Objective: Monitor the woman and reassess her vital signs.

- Determine the woman's BP, pulse, respirations, and FHR.
- Palpate the woman's fundus to assess for uterine contractions.
- Monitor the woman with an external fetal monitor for 20–30 minutes after the amniocentesis.

Rationale

Amniocentesis is usually performed laterally in the area of fetal small parts, where pockets of amniotic fluid are often seen. Real-time ultrasound will identify fetal parts and locate pockets of amniotic fluid.

Cleansing the woman's abdomen will decrease the incidence of infection.

It is important to determine if the fetus was inadvertently punctured.

- Determine a treatment course to counteract any supine hypotension and to increase venous return and cardiac output.
- Assess the woman's blood type and determine any need for Rh immune globulin.
- Have the woman lie on her left side.

Objective: Reassure the woman and provide self-care education.

- Instruct the woman to report any of the following side effects to her primary caretaker:
  a. Unusual fetal hyperactivity or lack of movement
  b. Vaginal discharge—clear drainage or bleeding
  c. Uterine contractions or abdominal pain
  d. Fever or chills

The woman will know how to recognize side effects or conditions that warrant further treatment.

- Encourage the woman to engage in only light activity for 24 hours.

A decrease in maternal activity will decrease uterine irritability and increase uteroplacental circulation.

- Encourage the woman to increase her fluid intake.

Increased hydration will replace the amniotic fluid through the uteroplacental circulation.

Objective: Complete the client record.

- Record the type of procedure, the date and time, and the name of the physician who performed the procedure.
- Record the maternal-fetus response, disposition of the specimen, and discharge teaching.

Provides a permanent record.

Assisting with a Pelvic Examination

Nursing Action

Objective: Provide a warm environment.

Turn on overhead heat lights, if available, or turn up the thermostat.

Objective: Assemble and prepare the equipment.

- Prepare and arrange the following items so that they are easily accessible:
  a. Vaginal specula of various sizes, warmed with water or on a heating pad prior to insertion
  b. Gloves
  c. Water-soluble lubricant
  d. Materials for Pap smear and cultures
  e. Good light source

- Do not use lubricant on the speculum before insertion.

Rationale

Warm environment promotes comfort.

Equipment organization facilitates the examination.

A warmed speculum assists in lubrication and facilitates initial insertion when culture and smears are taken.

Use of lubricant may alter findings or cultures.

Objective: Prepare the woman.

- Explain the procedure. If the woman has never had a pelvic examination, show her the equipment and explain the procedure before examination.

  Explanation of the procedure decreases anxiety.

- Instruct the woman to empty her bladder and to remove clothing below the waist. She may want to leave her shoes on.

  An empty bladder promotes comfort during internal examination. Some women feel more comfortable with shoes on, rather than supporting their weight with bare heels against cold stirrups.

- Give the woman a disposable drape or sheet to place on her lap. Encourage her to sit on the end of the examining table with the drape across her lap.

- Position the woman in the lithotomy position with her thighs flexed and adducted. Place her feet in the stirrups. Her buttocks should extend slightly beyond the end of the examining table.

- Drape the woman with the sheet, leaving a flap so the perineum can be exposed.

Objective: Provide support to the woman as the physician or nurse practitioner performs the examination.

- Explain each part of the examination as it is performed: inspection of external genitals, vagina, and cervix; bimanual examination of internal organs.

  Explanations promote relaxation.

(continued)

Assisting with a Pelvic Examination (continued)

Nursing Action

- Instruct the woman to relax and breathe slowly.
- Advise the woman when the speculum is about to be inserted and ask her to bear down.
- Lubricate the examiner's finger prior to bimanual examination.

Objective: Provide for the woman's comfort at the end of the examination.

- Move to the end of the examination table and face the woman's perineum. Cover the woman with the drape. Apply gentle pressure to the woman's knees and encourage her to move toward the head of the table. Offer your hand to the woman, remove her heels from the stirrups, and assist her to a sitting position. Be sure that she is not dizzy and that she is sitting or standing safely before you leave the room.
- Provide tissues to wipe lubricant from the perineum.
- Provide privacy while the woman dresses.

Rationale

When the speculum is inserted, the woman may feel intravaginal pressure. Bearing down helps open the vaginal orifice and relaxes the perineal muscles. Lubrication decreases friction and eases insertion.

The supine position may cause postural hypotension.

Upon assuming a sitting position, vaginal secretions along with lubricant may be discharged.

Auscultation of Fetal Heart Rate

Nursing Action	Rationale
Objective: Assemble the equipment.	
Obtain a fetoscope or a Doppler.	These devices amplify the fetal heart rate sounds.
Objective: Prepare the woman.	
• Explain the procedure, the indications for the procedure, and the information that will be obtained.	Explaining the procedure decreases anxiety and increases relaxation.
• Uncover the woman's abdomen.	
Objective: Use the fetoscope or Doppler as indicated and listen carefully for the FHR	
Objective: Check the woman's pulse, then count the FHR.	
• Check the woman's pulse against the fetal sounds you hear. If the rates are the same, you have probably located maternal pulses and you need to readjust the fetoscope or ultrasound device.	

(continued)

Auscultation of Fetal Heart Rate (continued)

Nursing Action

- If the rates are not similar, count the FHR for 1 full minute. Note that the fetal heart has a double rhythm and just one sound is counted.
- If you do not find the FHR, move the fetoscope or ultrasound device laterally.
- Explain to the parents what the FHR is and offer to help them listen if they would like to.

Objective: Systematically evaluate the FHR.

Auscultate between, during, and for 30 seconds following a uterine contraction (UC).

AWHONN (1998) Frequency Recommendations

- Low-risk women: every 1 hour in the latent phase, every 30 minutes in the active phase, and every 15 minutes in the second stage.
- High-risk women: every 30 minutes in the latent phase, every 15 minutes in the active phase, and every 5 minutes in the second stage.

Rationale

This evaluation provides the opportunity to assess the fetal status and response to the labor process.

Objective: Record the information on the woman's chart.

Document FHR data (rate and rhythm), characteristics of uterine activity, and any actions taken as a result of the FHR. Complete documentation is mandatory.

Sample recordings follow.

Sample Documentation

Entry documenting FHR, rhythm, and response to the labor process:

1-1-02   FHR 140 by auscultation, regular rhythm, Maternal pulse 78.

0730   UC q3min × 60 sec strong. No increase or decrease in FHR noted during or following UC. J Smith RN

Entry documenting FHR, response to UC, nursing intervention, and fetal response:

1-1-02   FHR 136 by auscultation with slowing to 130 bpm noted during the acme of UC and for

0730   10 sec following the UC, STV present, LTV average. Client turned to left side. Maternal pulse 80, FHR 140, regular rhythm with no decrease during or following the next two UC. UC q3min × 60 sec, strong, J Smith RN

(continued)

Auscultation of Fetal Heart Rate (continued)

Nursing Action

Using a Fetoscope or a Doppler Ultrasound Device

The Fetoscope

The fetoscope is an older assessment tool; however, some clinicians prefer it because it is "natural" and does not rely on ultrasound.

To use the fetoscope:

- Place the fetoscope earpieces in your ears; use the handpiece to position the bell of the fetoscope on the mother's abdomen.

- Place the diaphragm halfway between the umbilicus and symphysis and in the midline. *You are most likely to hear the FHR in this area.*

- Without touching the fetoscope, listen carefully for the FHR.

Rationale

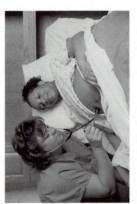

The nurse holds the fetoscope as she places it against the maternal abdomen and then removes her fingers from the fetoscope while counting the fetal heartbeats.

The Doppler

To use the Doppler:

- Place ultrasonic gel on the diaphragm of the Doppler. Gel is used to maintain contact with the maternal abdomen and enhances conduction of ultrasound.

- Place the diaphragm on the woman's abdomen halfway between the umbilicus and symphysis and in the midline. You are most likely to hear the FHR in this area.

- Listen carefully for the FHR.

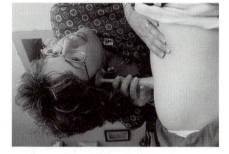

The Penar fetoscope can be easily used in outpatient or community settings.

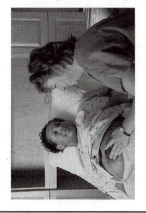

When the fetal heart rate is picked up by the electronic monitor, the sound of the heartbeat can be heard by all persons in the room.

Electronic Fetal Monitoring

Nursing Action	Rationale
Objective: Prepare the woman.	
Explain the procedure, the indications for the procedure, and the information that will be obtained.	Explaining the procedure decreases anxiety and increases relaxation.
Objective: Place the external fetal monitor.	
• Turn on the monitor.	
• Place two elastic belts around the woman's abdomen.	
• Place the "toco" over the uterine fundus off the midline on the area palpated to be most firm and secure it with a belt so it fits snugly.	The uterine fundus is the area of greatest contractility.
• Note the UC tracing. The resting tone tracing (without uterine contraction) should be recording on the 10 or 15 mm Hg pressure line. Adjust the line to reflect that reading.	If the tracing is on the zero line, there may be a constant grinding noise.
• Apply ultrasonic gel to the diaphragm of the ultrasound transducer.	Ultrasound gel is used to maintain contact with the maternal abdomen. The ultrasonic beam is directed toward the fetal heart.
• Place the diaphragm on the maternal abdomen in the midline between the umbilicus and the symphysis pubis.	

- Listen for the FHR, which will have a whiplike sound. When the FHR is located, attach the elastic belt snugly. Firm contact is necessary to maintain a continuous tracing.

Objective: Identify the tracing.

Place the following information on the beginning of the fetal monitor paper: date, time, client name, gravida, para, membrane status, physician or CNM name. *Note:* Each birthing area may have specific guidelines regarding additional information to include.

This ensures accurate identification.

Objective: Evaluate the EFM tracing.

See the material that follows for evaluation guidelines.

Objective: Report and record your findings.

Reporting provides a permanent record.

Sample Documentation

Entry documenting reassuring FHR characteristics and response to UCs:

1-1-02   FHR BL 135–140. STV and LTV present. Two acceleration of 20 bpm × 20 sec with

0700   fetal movement in 10 min. UC q3min × 50–60 sec of moderate intensity by palpation, resting tone soft. No decelerations noted. B Burch, RNC

(continued)

Electronic Fetal Monitoring (continued)

Nursing Action

Sample Documentation continued

Entry documenting FHR, variability, response of FHR to UC, the intervention used, and subsequent positive fetal response to the intervention.

1-1-02   FHR BL 135–140. STV and LTV present. Late decelerations noted with decrease of FHR

0730   to 130 bpm for 20 sec. UC q3min × 50–60 sec of moderate intensity by palpation. Client turned to left side. No further deceleration with three subsequent UCs. Two accelerations of 20 bpm × 20 sec noted with fetal movement. Client instructed to remain on left side. B Burch, RNC

Guidelines for Evaluating the EFM

Evaluating the EFM tracing provides an opportunity to assess the fetal status and response to the labor process. The presence of reassuring characteristics is associated with good fetal outcome. Rapid identification of nonreassuring characteristics allows prompt interventions and the opportunity to determine the fetal response to the interventions.

Rationale

For high-risk women, AWHONN (1998) recommends evaluating the EFM tracing every 15 minutes in the first stage and every 5 minutes in the second stage; for low-risk women, every 15–30 minutes in the first stage and every 5–15 minutes in the second stage (as long as the FHR has reassuring characteristics). The time interval for evaluation needs to be shortened if any nonreassuring characteristics occur.

Evaluating Lochia After Birth

Nursing Action

Objective: Prepare the woman.

Explain the procedure, the reason for performing the procedure, and the information that will be obtained.

Objective: Obtain and evaluate maternal vital signs.

Assess maternal temperature, blood pressure, and pulse.

Objective: Accurately evaluate the amount of lochia after birth.

- Don disposable gloves.
- Lower the perineal pad so that you can visualize the amount of lochia.
- Palpate the uterine fundus, located in the midline at the umbilicus or one to two finger breadths below the umbilicus, by placing one hand on the fundus and the other hand just over the symphysis pubis and pressing downward. Use your other hand to palpate the fundus.

Rationale

Explaining the procedure decreases anxiety and increases relaxation.

This provides information regarding the woman's physiologic status.

Universal precautions and body substance isolation require use of gloves when exposed to body secretions.

Downward pressure exerted just above the symphysis pubis will prevent excessive downward movement of the uterus during assessment.

(continued)

Evaluating Lochia After Birth (continued)

Nursing Action

- Determine the firmness of the fundus.
- If the fundus is boggy, massage by rubbing in a circular motion.
- Evaluate the color and amount of lochia and observe for clots.

Lochia Evaluation Guidelines

Small: Smaller than a 4-in stain on the pad; 10 to 25 mL
Moderate: Smaller than a 6-in stain; 25 to 50 mL
Large: Larger than a 6-in stain; 50 to 80 mL

If blood loss exceeds the above guidelines, weigh the perineal pads and the Chux to estimate the blood loss more accurately (1 g = 1 mL).

Rationale

The uterus must remain firmly contracted to prevent excessive blood loss. Manual pressure stimulates uterine contractions.

Weighing the pads and Chux can provide important information. Because some blood loss is normal, care providers may not otherwise detect excessive blood loss.

Performing a Heel Stick on a Newborn

Nursing Action

Objective: Assemble the equipment.

- Microlancet (do not use a needle)
- Alcohol swabs
- 2×2 sterile gauze squares
- Small bandage
- Transfer pipette
- Glucose reagent strips or reflectance meters
- Gloves

Objective: Prepare the infant's heel for the procedure.

- Use a warm, wet wrap or specially designed chemical heat pad to warm the infant's heel for 5–10 seconds to facilitate blood flow.
- Select a clear, previously unpunctured site.
- Clean the site by rubbing vigorously with 70% isopropyl alcohol swab, followed by a dry gauze square.
- Blot the site dry completely before lancing.

Rationale

Equipment organization facilitates the procedure. A needle may nick the periosteum.

Gloves are used to implement universal precautions and prevent nosocomial infections.

The selection of a previously unpunctured site minimizes the risk of infection and excessive scar formation. Friction produces local heat, which aids vasodilation. Alcohol is irritating to injured tissue, and it may also produce hemolysis.

(continued)

Performing a Heel Stick on a Newborn (continued)

Nursing Action

Objective: Lance the infant's heel and ensure accurate blood sampling. See the step-by-step instructions that follow.

Objective: Prevent excessive bleeding.

- Apply a folded gauze square to the puncture site and secure it firmly with a bandage.
- Check the puncture site frequently for the first hour after sampling.

Objective: Record the findings on the infant's chart.

Report immediately any results under 45 mg/dL or over 175 mg/dL for glucose.

Performing the Heel Stick

The infant's lateral heel is the site of choice because it precludes damaging the posterior tibial nerve and artery, plantar artery, and the important longitudinally oriented fat pad of the heel, which in later years could impede walking. This is especially

Rationale

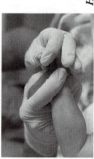

Recording the results helps identify possible complications.

Heel sticks.

important for infants undergoing multiple heel stick procedures. Toes are acceptable sites if necessary.

Lancing the Heel

- Grasp the infant's lower leg and foot so as to impede venous return slightly. This will facilitate extraction of the blood sample.
- With a quick, piercing motion, puncture the lateral heel with a microlancet. Be careful not to puncture too deeply. Optimal penetration is 4 mm.

Collecting the Blood Sample

- Use transfer pipette to place drop of blood on glucose reflectance meter.
- Use capillary tube for hematocrit testing.

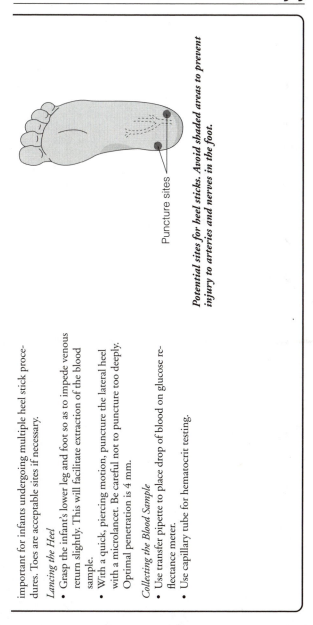

Puncture sites

Potential sites for heel sticks. Avoid shaded areas to prevent injury to arteries and nerves in the foot.

Performing an Intrapartal Vaginal Examination

Nursing Action	Rationale
Objective: Assemble the equipment.	
Prepare and arrange the following items so they are easily accessible:	Organizing the equipment facilitates the examination.
• Clean disposable gloves	If membranes are ruptured, sterile disposable gloves are used to decrease the chance of introducing bacteria during the examination. When membranes are intact, clean disposable gloves may be used.
• Lubricant	
• Nitrazine test tape	
• Slide	
• Sterile cotton-tipped swab (Q-Tip)	
Objective: Prepare the woman.	
• Explain the procedure, the indications for the exam, what the exam may feel like, and that it may cause discomfort. In-	By explaining the procedure, the nurse decreases anxiety and increases relaxation.
• Assess for latex allergies.	Select nonlatex gloves if woman is allergic.
• Position the woman with her thighs flexed and abducted. Instruct her to put the heels of her feet together. Drape the woman with a sheet, leaving a flap to access the perineum.	Position provides access to the vulvar area.
	The drape provides privacy.

- Encourage the woman to relax her muscles and legs.
- Inform the woman prior to touching her. Use gentleness.

Objective: Test for amniotic fluid leakage if indicated.

If fluid leakage has been reported or noted, use Nitrazine test tape and Q-Tip with slide for fern test before performing the exam.

- Fern test is done by inserting the swab in the pooling of fluid in the posterior vagina and applying the fluid to a slide.

Objective: Use aseptic technique during the exam.

- Pull glove onto dominant hand.
- Using your gloved hand, position the hand with the wrist straight and the elbow tilted downward. Insert your well-lubricated second and index fingers of the gloved hand into the vagina until they touch the cervix. Use care when positioning your hand.
- If the woman verbalizes discomfort, acknowledge it and apologize.

Objective: Determine the status of labor progress.

- Perform the vaginal examination during and between contractions.

Relaxation decreases muscle tension and increases comfort.
This action communicates regard for the woman and her privacy.

As long as lubricant has not been used, Nitrazine tape registers a change in pH if amniotic fluid is present.
Digital exam may be deferred if the woman has ruptured membranes and is not actively laboring (AAP & ACOG, 1997).

If sterile exam is needed, both hands will be gloved with sterile gloves.
This positioning allows the fingertips to point toward the umbilicus and find the cervix.

This validates the woman's feelings and helps her feel more in control.

Cervical dilatation, effacement, and fetal station are affected by the presence of a contraction.

(continued)

Performing an Intrapartal Vaginal Examination (continued)

Nursing Action	Rationale
Objective: Identify the amount of cervical dilatation and effacement.	
• Palpate for the opening, or a depression, in the cervix. Estimate the diameter of the depression to identify the amount of dilatation.	Allows determination of effacement and dilatation.
Objective: Determine the status of the fetal membranes.	
• Observe for expression of amniotic fluid.	If fluid is expressed, test for amniotic fluid.

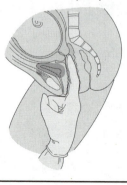

To gauge cervical dilatation, the nurse places the index and middle fingers against the cervix and determines the size of the opening. Before labor begins, the cervix is long (approximately 2.5 cm), the sides feel thick, and the cervical canal is closed, so an examining finger cannot be inserted. During labor, the cervix begins to dilate, and the size of the opening progresses from 1 cm to 10 cm in diameter.

Objective: Palpate the presenting part.

Provides information regarding fetal descent and cardinal movements.

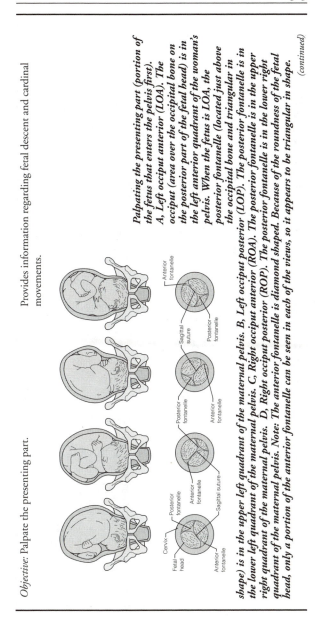

shape) is in the upper left quadrant of the maternal pelvis. B, Left occiput posterior (LOP). The posterior fontanelle is in the lower left quadrant of the maternal pelvis. C, Right occiput anterior (ROA). The posterior fontanelle is in the upper right quadrant of the maternal pelvis. D, Right occiput posterior (ROP). The posterior fontanelle is in the lower right quadrant of the maternal pelvis. Note: The anterior fontanelle is diamond shaped. Because of the roundness of the fetal head, only a portion of the anterior fontanelle can be seen in each of the views.

Palpating the presenting part (portion of the fetus that enters the pelvis first).
A, Left occiput anterior (LOA). The occiput (area over the occipital bone on the posterior part of the fetal head) is in the left anterior quadrant of the woman's pelvis. When the fetus is LOA, the posterior fontanelle (located just above the occipital bone and triangular in shape) is in the upper left quadrant of the maternal pelvis.

(continued)

Performing an Intrapartal Vaginal Examination (continued)

Nursing Action

Objective: Assess the fetal descent.

- Assess the station; identify the position of the posterior fontanelle.

Rationale

Provides information regarding fetal descent and position.

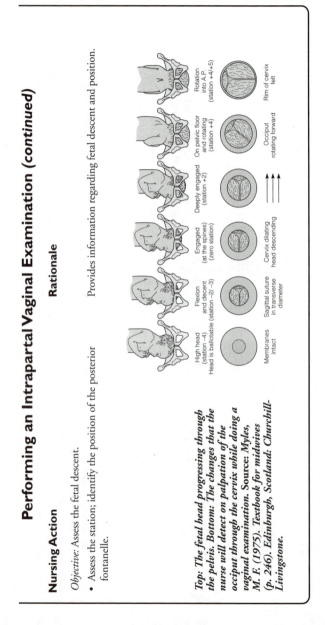

High head (station −4) Head is ballottable (station −2/ −3)

Flexion and descent (station −2/ −3)

Engaged (at the spines) (zero station)

Deeply engaged (station +2)

On pelvic floor and rotating (station +4)

Rotation into A.P (station +4/+5)

Membranes intact

Sagittal suture in transverse diameter

Cervix dilating head descending

Occiput rotating forward

Rim of cervix felt

Top: The fetal head progressing through the pelvis. Bottom: The changes that the nurse will detect on palpation of the occiput through the cervix while doing a vaginal examination. Source: Myles, M. F. (1975). Textbook for midwives (p. 246). Edinburgh, Scotland: Churchill-Livingstone.

Performing Gavage Feeding

Nursing Action

Objective: Assemble and prepare the equipment.

- No. 5 or no. 8 Fr. feeding tube. See the material that follows for guidelines for choosing tube size. Equipment organization facilitates the procedure.
- 10–30 mL syringe, for aspirating stomach contents
- 1/4-in. paper tape, to mark the tube for insertion depth and to secure the catheter during feeding
- Stethoscope, for auscultating the rush of air into the stomach when testing the tube placement
- Appropriate formula
- Small cup of sterile water to test for tube placement and to act as lubricant

Objective: Explain the procedure to the parents.

Objective: Insert the tube accurately into the stomach.

- See the material below for gavage feeding guidelines.

Rationale

Equipment organization facilitates the procedure.

(continued)

Performing Gavage Feeding (continued)

Nursing Action	Rationale
Objective: Maximize the feeding pleasure of the infant.	Feeding time is important to the infant's tactile sensory input.
• Whenever possible, hold the infant during gavage feeding. If it is too awkward to hold the infant during feeding, be sure to take time for holding after the feeding.	Sucking during feeding comforts and relaxes the infant, making the formula flow more easily. Infants can lose their sucking reflexes when fed by gavage for long periods.
• Offer a pacifier to the infant during the feeding.	

Gavage Feeding Guidelines

Choosing a Catheter Size

When choosing the catheter size, consider the size of the infant, the area of insertion (oral or nasal), and the desired rate of flow. The size of the catheter will influence the rate of flow.

The very small infant (less than 1600 g) requires a 5 Fr. feeding tube; an infant greater than 1600 g may tolerate a larger tube.

Orogastric insertion is preferable to nasogastric because most infants are obligatory nose breathers. If nasogastric is used, a 5 Fr. catheter should be used to minimize airway obstruction.

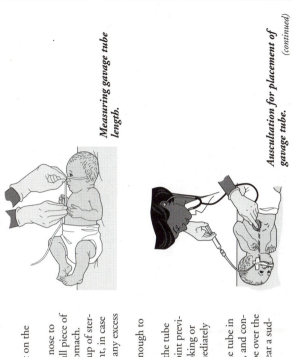

Measuring gavage tube length.

Auscultation for placement of gavage tube.

(continued)

Inserting and Checking the Tube

- Elevate the head of the bed and position the infant on the back or side to allow easy passage of the tube.

- Measure the distance from the tip of the ear to the nose to the xiphoid process and mark the point with a small piece of paper tape to ensure enough tubing to enter the stomach.

- If inserting the tube nasally, lubricate the tip in a cup of sterile water. Use water instead of an oil-based lubricant, in case the tube is inadvertently passed into a lung. Shake any excess drops to prevent aspiration.

- If inserting the tube orally, the oral secretions are enough to lubricate the tube adequately.

- Stabilize the infant's head with one hand and pass the tube via the mouth (or nose) into the stomach to the point previously marked. If the infant begins coughing or choking or becomes cyanotic or phonic, remove the tube immediately because the tube has probably entered the trachea.

- If no respiratory distress is apparent, lightly tape the tube in position, draw up 0.5–1.0 mL of air in the syringe, and connect the syringe to the tubing. Place the stethoscope over the epigastric area and briskly inject the air. You will hear a sudden air rush as the air enters the stomach.

Performing Gavage Feeding (continued)

Nursing Action

- Aspirate the stomach contents with the syringe and note the amount, color, and consistency to evaluate the infant's feeding tolerance. Return the residual to the stomach unless you are asked to discard it. It is usually not discarded because of the potential for electrolyte imbalance.

- If the aspirated contents contain only a clear fluid or mucus and if it is unclear whether the tube is in the stomach, test the aspirate for pH. Stomach aspirate has a pH between 1 and 3.

Administering the Feeding

- Hold the infant for feeding or position the infant on the right side to decrease the risk of aspiration in case of emesis during feeding.

- Separate the syringe from the tube, remove the plunger from the barrel, reconnect the barrel to the tube, and pour the formula into the syringe.

- Elevate the syringe 6–8 in. over the infant's head and allow the formula to flow by gravity at a slow, even rate. You may

need to initiate the flow of formula by inserting the plunger of the syringe into the barrel just until you see formula enter the feeding tube. Do not use pressure.

- Regulate the rate to prevent sudden stomach distension, leading to vomiting and aspiration. Continue adding formula to the syringe until the infant has absorbed the desired volume.

Clearing and Removing the Tube

- Clear the tubing with 2–3 mL sterile water or with air. This ensures that the infant has received all of the formula. If the tube is going to be left in place, clearing it will decrease the risk of clogging and bacterial growth in the tube.

- To remove the tube, loosen the tape, fold the tube over on itself, and quickly withdraw the tube in one smooth motion to minimize the potential for fluid aspiration as the tube passes the epiglottis. If the tube is to be left in, position it so that the infant is unable to remove it. Replace the tube every 24 hours.

Performing Nasal Pharyngeal Suctioning

Nursing Action

Objective: Clear secretions from the newborn's nose or oropharynx if respirations are depressed or if amniotic fluid was meconium stained.

- Tighten the lid on the DeLee mucus trap or other suction device collection bottle.
- Connect one end of the DeLee tubing to low suction.
- Insert the other end of the tubing 3 to 5 in into the newborn's nose or mouth.

Rationale

This avoids spillage of secretions and prevents air from leaking out of the lid.

DeLee mucus trap.

(continued)

Performing Nasal Pharyngeal Suctioning (continued)

Nursing Action

- Continue suction as you remove the tube.
- Continue to reinsert the tube and provide suction for as long as fluid is aspirated. *Note: Excessive suctioning can cause vagal stimulation, which decreases heart rate.*
- If it is necessary to pass the tube into the newborn's stomach to remove meconium secretions that the newborn swallowed before birth, insert the tube into the newborn's mouth and then into the stomach. Provide suction and continue suction as you remove the tube.

Objective: Record relevant information on the newborn's chart.

Document completion of the procedure and the amount and type of secretions.

Rationale

This avoids repositing secretions in the newborn's nasopharynx.

This provides documentation of intervention and status at birth.

Thermoregulation of the Newborn

Nursing Action

Objective: Prepare the warming equipment.

- Prewarm the incubator or radiant warmer. Make sure warmed towels and/or lightweight blankets are available.
- Maintain the birthing room at 22°C (71°F), with a relative humidity of 60%–65%.

Objective: Establish a stable temperature after birth.

- Wipe the newborn free of blood and excessive vernix, especially from the head, with prewarmed towels.
- Place the newborn under the radiant warmer.
- Wrap the newborn in a prewarmed blanket and transfer the newborn to the mother.
- Place the infant skin to skin on the mother's chest under a warmed blanket.

Rationale

The change from a warm, moist intrauterine environment to a cool, dry, drafty environment stresses the newborn's immature thermoregulation mechanisms.

This prevents loss of body heat from a large surface area through evaporation.

The radiant warmer creates a heat-gaining environment.

Use of the prewarmed blanket reduces convective heat loss and facilitates maternal-infant contact without compromising the newborn's thermoregulation.

Skin-to-skin contact with the mother or father helps maintain the newborn's temperature.

(continued)

Thermoregulation of the Newborn (continued)

Nursing Action

Objective: Maintain a stable infant temperature.

- Diaper the newborn and place a stocking hat on his or her head. Place the newborn uncovered (except for diaper and hat) under the radiant warmer.

- Tape a servocontrol probe on the newborn's anterior abdominal wall, with the metal side next to the skin, and cover the probe with an aluminum heat deflector patch.

- Turn the heater to servocontrol mode so that the abdominal skin is maintained at 36.5°C–37°C (97.5–98.6°F).

- Monitor the newborn's axillary and skin probe temperature per institution's protocol.

- When the newborn's temperature reaches 37°C (98.6°F), remove the infant from the radiant warmer and place a T-shirt, diaper, and stocking hat on the newborn.

- Double wrap (two blankets) the newborn and place the newborn in an open crib.

- Recheck the newborn's axillary temperature in 1 hour.

Rationale

Radiant heat warms the outer surface skin, so the skin needs to be exposed.

Do not place over ribs. The aluminum cover prevents heating of the probe directly and overheating the infant.

The temperature indicator on the radiant warmer continually displays the newborn's probe temperature, so the axillary temperature is checked to ensure that the machine accurately reports the newborn's temperature.

It is important to monitor the infant's ability to maintain its own thermoregulation.

Objective: Rewarm the newborn gradually if temperature drops below 36.1°C (97°F).

- Access axillary temperature frequently, per agency routine, usually every 2–4 hours.

  Frequent assessment may detect hypothermia, which predisposes the newborn to cold stress.

- If the newborn needs rewarming, place the newborn (unclothed except for diaper) under the radiant warmer with a servocontrol probe on the anterior abdominal wall.
- Gradually rewarm back to normal temperature.
- Recheck the newborn's temperature in 30 minutes, then hourly. When the temperature reaches 37°C (98.6°F), remove the newborn from the radiant heater, dress the newborn, double wrap, and place in the open crib. Recheck the temperature in 1 hour.

  Rapid heating can lead to hyperthermia, which is associated with apnea, increased insensible water loss, and increased metabolic rate.

Objective: Prevent drops in the newborn's temperature.

The nurse carries out the following activities:

- Keep the newborn's clothing and bedding dry.
- Double wrap the newborn and put a stocking hat on him or her.
- Use the radiant warmer during procedures.
- Reduce the newborn's exposure to drafts.

(continued)

Thermoregulation of the Newborn (continued)

Nursing Action

- Warm objects that will come in contact with the newborn (eg, stethoscopes).
- Encourage the mother to snuggle with the newborn under blankets or breastfeed the newborn with hat and light cover on.

Rationale

Maternal-Child Health Care

American Academy of Pediatrics
(AAP)
Elk Grove Village, IL 60007
1-847-434-4000
Fax 1-847-434-8000
http://www.aap.org

Association of Women's Health,
Obstetrics and Neonatal
Nurses (AWHONN)
Washington, DC 20036
1-800-673-8499
Fax 1-202-728-0575
http://www.awhonn.org

American College of Obstetricians and Gynecologists
(ACOG)
Washington, DC 20090-6920
1-202-863-2518
Fax 1-202-479-6826
http://www.acog.org

Maternal and Child Health
Bureau
Health and Human Services
Rockville, MD 20857
1-301-443-2170
Fax 1-301-443-1797
http://www.mchb.hrsa.gov

National Child Care Information Center
243 Church Street NW, 2nd
Floor
Vienna, VA 22180
1-800-616-2242
Fax 1-800-716-2242
http://NCCIC.org

National Maternal and Child
Health Clearinghouse (Circle Solutions, Inc.)
(provides information and pub-
lications regarding maternal-
child health, nutrition,
pregnancy, etc)
Vienna, VA 22182
1-703-821-8955
Fax 1-703-821-2098
http://www.circsol.com

Multicultural Resources

AT&T Language Line
(24-hour access to interpreters
who speak over 100
languages)
1-800-752-6096

African Americans

Black Women's Health Council
P.O. Box 31089
Capitol Heights, MD 20731
1-301-808-0786
Fax 1-301-808-0963

National Black Women's Health
Project
1211 Connecticut Avenue NW,
Suite 310
Washington, DC 20036
1-202-835-0117
Fax 1-202-833-8790

Asian Americans

Asian Health Services
Oakland, CA 94607
1-510-986-6800
Fax 1-510-986-6896
http://www.ahschc.org

Asian and Pacific Islander American Health Forum, Inc.
San Francisco, CA 94102
1-415-954-9988
Fax 1-415-954-9999
http://www.apiahf.org

Hispanic/Latino Americans

National Coalition of Hispanic Health and Human Services Organizations (COSSMHO)
Washington, DC 20036-1401
1-202-387-5000
Fax 1-202-797-4353
http://www.hispanichealth.org

Native Americans

Indian Health Service (IHS)
Health Resources and Services Administration
Department of Health and Human Services
Rockville, MD 20857
1-301-443-3593
Fax 1-301-443-0507
http://www.ihis.gov

Specific Health Conditions

Alcohol and Drug Abuse
National Clearinghouse for Alcohol and Drug Information
Rockville, MD 20847-2345
1-800-729-6686
Fax 1-301-468-6433
http://www.health.org

HIV-AIDS Infections

AIDS National Interface Network
110 Maryland Avenue, NE, Suite 504
Washington, DC 20002
1-202-546-0807
Fax 1-202-546-5103

National Aids Hotline
1-800-342-AIDS
http://www.ashastd.org/nah

Sexually Transmitted Diseases

Sexuality Information and Education Council of the United States
New York, NY 10036
1-212-819-9770
Fax 1-212-819-9776
http://www.siecus.org

Women's Health

National Resource Center on Women and Aids
Center for Women Policy Studies
Washington, DC 20036
1-202-872-1770
Fax 1-202-296-8962

Workplace Health Promotion

Association for Worksite Health Promotion
Northbrook, IL 60062
1-847-480-9574
Fax 1-847-480-9282
http://ww.awhp.org

Common Abbreviations in Maternal-Newborn Nursing

AC	Abdominal circumference
accel	Acceleration of fetal heart rate
AFAFP	Amniotic fluid alpha fetoprotein
AFP	α-fetoprotein
AFV	Amniotic fluid volume
AGA	Average for gestational age
AMOL	Active management of labor
AOP	Apnea of prematurity *or* Anemia of prematurity
ARBOW	Artificial rupture of bag of waters
AROM	Artificial rupture of membranes
BAT	Brown adipose tissue (brown fat)
BL	Baseline (fetal heart rate baseline)
BOW	Bag of waters
BPD	Biparietal diameter *or* Bronchopulmonary dysplasia
bpm	Beats per minute
BPP	Biophysical profile
BSE	Breast self-examination
BSST	Breast self-stimulation test
CC	Chest circumference *or* Cord compression
C–H	Crown-to-heel length
CID	Cytomegalic inclusion disease
CMV	Cytomegalovirus
CNM	Certified nurse-midwife
CPD	Cephalopelvic disproportion
CRL	Crown-rump length

C/S	Cesarean section or (C-section)
CST	Contraction stress test
CVS	Chorionic villus sampling
decels	Deceleration of fetal heart rate
DIC	Disseminated intravascular coagulation
dil	Dilatation
DTR	Deep tendon reflexes
ECHMO	Extracorporeal membrane oxygenator
EDB	Estimated date of birth
EDC	Estimated date of confinement
EFM	Electronic fetal monitoring
epis	Episiotomy
FAE	Fetal alcohol effects
FAS	Fetal alcohol syndrome
FB	Finger breadth
FBM	Fetal breathing movements
FBS	Fetal blood sample *or* Fasting blood sugar test
FHR	Fetal heart rate
FHT	Fetal heart tones
FL	Femur length
FM	Fetal movement
FSH	Follicle-stimulating hormone
G or grav	Gravida
GDM	Gestational diabetes mellitus
GERD	Gastric esophageal reflux disease
GTPAL	Gravida, term, preterm, abortion, living children
HA	Head-abdominal
HAI	Hemagglutination inhibition
HC	Head compression
hCG	Human chorionic gonadotrophin
hCS	Human chorionic somatomammotrophin (same as hPL)
HMD	Hyaline membrane disease
hPL	Human placental lactogen
HVH	Herpesvirus hominis
IDDM	Insulin-dependent diabetes mellitus
IDM	Infant of a diabetic mother
IUD	Intrauterine device
IUFD	Intrauterine fetal death

IUGR	Intrauterine growth retardation or restriction
LADA	Left-acromion-dorsal-anterior
LADP	Left-acromion-dorsal-posterior
LBW	Low birth weight
LDR	Labor, delivery, and recovery room
LGA	Large for gestational age
LMA	Left-mentum-anterior
LML	Left mediolateral (episiotomy)
LMP	Last menstrual period *or* Left-mentum-posterior
LMT	Left-mentum-transverse
LOA	Left-occiput-anterior
LOF	Low outlet forceps
LOP	Left-occiput-posterior
LOT	Left-occiput-transverse
L/S	Lecithin/sphingomyelin
LSA	Left-sacrum-anterior
LSP	Left-sacrum-posterior
LST	Left-sacrum-transverse
LTV	Long-term variability
MAS	Meconium aspiration syndrome
mec	Meconium
mec st	Meconium stain
ML	Midline (episiotomy)
MSAFP	Maternal serum alpha-fetoprotein
multip	Multipara
NEC	Necrotizing enterocolitis
NIDDM	Non-insulin-dependent diabetes mellitus
NSCST	Nipple stimulation contraction stress test
NST	Nonstress test *or* Nonshivering thermogenesis
NTD	Neural tube defects
NTE	Neutral thermal environment
OA	Occiput anterior
OF	Occipitofrontal diameter of fetal head
OFC	Occipitofrontal circumference
OM	Occipitomental (diameter)
OP	Occiput posterior
P	Para
Pap smear	Papanicolaou smear
PDA	Patent ductus arteriosus

PEEP	Positive end-expiratory pressure
PG	Phosphatidylglycerol *or* Prostaglandin
PI	Phosphatidylinositol
PIH	Pregnancy-induced hypertension
Pit	Pitocin
PKU	Phenylketonuria
PPHN	Persistent pulmonary hypertension
Preemie	Premature infant
Primip	Primipara
PROM	Premature rupture of membranes
PUBS	Percutaneous umbilical blood sampling
RADA	Right-acromion-dorsal-anterior
RADP	Right-acromion-dorsal-posterior
RDS	Respiratory distress syndrome
RIA	Radioimmune assay
RLF	Retrolental fibroplasia
RMA	Right-mentum-anterior
RMP	Right-mentum-posterior
RMT	Right-mentum-transverse
ROA	Right-occiput-anterior
ROM	Rupture of membranes
ROP	Right-occiput-posterior *or* Retinopathy of prematurity
ROT	Right-occiput-transverse
RSA	Right-sacrum-anterior
RSP	Right-sacrum-posterior
RST	Right-sacrum-transverse
SET	Surrogate embryo transfer
SGA	Small for gestational age
SIDS	Sudden infant death syndrome
SOB	Suboccipitobregmatic diameter *or* Shortness of breath
SRBOW	Spontaneous rupture of bag of waters
SROM	Spontaneous rupture of the membranes
STI	Sexually transmitted infection
STS	Serologic test for syphilis *or* Sexually transmitted serology
STV	Short-term variability
TC	Thoracic circumference
TCM	Transcutaneous monitoring

TDI	Therapeutic donor insemination
TOL	Trail of labor
TORCH	Toxoplasmosis, rubella, cytomegalovirus, herpesvirus hominis type 2
ū	Umbilicus
UA	Uterine activity
UAC	Umbilical artery catheter
UAU	Uterine activity units
UC	Uterine contraction
UPI	Uteroplacental insufficiency
U/S	Ultrasound
VBAC	Vaginal birth after cesarean
VDRL	Venereal Disease Research Laboratories
VLBW	Very low birth weight
WIC	Supplemental food program for Women, Infants, and Children
ZIFT	Zygote intrafallopian transfer

Appendix B

Conversion of Pounds and Ounces to Grams

Conversion of Pounds and Ounces to Grams

POUNDS	OUNCES 0	1	2	3	4	5	6	7	8	9	10	11	12	13	14	15
0		28	57	85	113	142	170	198	227	255	283	312	340	369	397	425
1	454	482	510	539	567	595	624	652	680	709	737	765	794	822	850	879
2	907	936	964	992	1021	1049	1077	1106	1134	1162	1191	1219	1247	1276	1304	1332
3	1361	1389	1417	1446	1474	1503	1531	1559	1588	1616	1644	1673	1701	1729	1758	1786
4	1814	1843	1871	1899	1928	1956	1984	2013	2041	2070	2098	2126	2155	2183	2211	2240
5	2268	2296	2325	2353	2381	2410	2438	2466	2495	2523	2551	2580	2608	2637	2665	2693
6	2722	2750	2778	2807	2835	2863	2892	2920	2948	2977	3005	3033	3062	3090	3118	3147
7	3175	3203	3232	3260	3289	3317	3345	3374	3402	3430	3459	3487	3515	3544	3572	3600
8	3629	3657	3685	3714	3742	3770	3799	3827	3856	3884	3912	3941	3969	3997	4026	4054
9	4082	4111	4139	4167	4196	4224	4252	4281	4309	4337	4366	4394	4423	4451	4479	4508
10	4536	4564	4593	4621	4649	4678	4706	4734	4763	4791	4819	4848	4876	4904	4933	4961
11	4990	5018	5046	5075	5103	5131	5160	5188	5216	5245	5273	5301	5330	5358	5386	5415
12	5443	5471	5500	5528	5557	5585	5613	5642	5670	5698	5727	5755	5783	5812	5840	5868
13	5897	5925	5953	5982	6010	6038	6067	6095	6123	6152	6180	6209	6237	6265	6294	6322
14	6350	6379	6407	6435	6464	6492	6520	6549	6577	6605	6634	6662	6690	6719	6747	6776
15	6804	6832	6860	6889	6917	6945	6973	7002	7030	7059	7087	7115	7144	7172	7201	7228
16	7257	7286	7313	7342	7371	7399	7427	7456	7484	7512	7541	7569	7597	7626	7654	7682
17	7711	7739	7768	7796	7824	7853	7881	7909	7938	7966	7994	8023	8051	8079	8108	8136
18	8165	8192	8221	8249	8278	8306	8335	8363	8391	8420	8448	8476	8504	8533	8561	8590
19	8618	8646	8675	8703	8731	8760	8788	8816	8845	8873	8902	8930	8958	8987	9015	9043
20	9072	9100	9128	9157	9185	9213	9242	9270	9298	9327	9355	9383	9412	9440	9469	9497
21	9525	9554	9582	9610	9639	9667	9695	9724	9752	9780	9809	9837	9865	9894	9922	9950
22	9979	10007	10036	10064	10092	10120	10149	10177	10206	10234	10262	10291	10319	10347	10376	10404

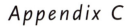
Appendix C

Cervical Dilatation
Assessment Aid

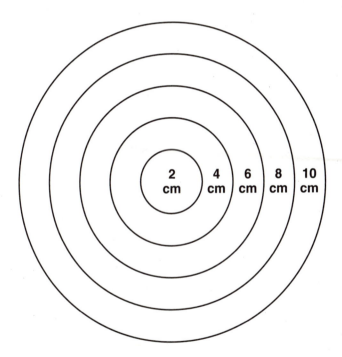

2 cm 4 cm 6 cm 8 cm 10 cm

Appendix D

Actions and Effects of Selected Drugs During Breastfeeding*

Anticoagulants

Coumarin derivatives (warfarin, dicumarol): Relatively safe to use; only small amount in breast milk; check PTT

Heparin: Does not cross into breast milk; check PTT

Phenindione (Hedulin): Passes easily into breast milk; neonate may have increased prothrombin time and PTT

Anticonvulsants

Phenytoin (Dilantin), phenobarbital: Generally considered safe; if high doses of phenobarbital are ingested, may cause drowsiness; short-acting phenobarbiturates (secobarbital) preferred, because they appear in lower concentration in milk

Magnesium sulfate: Lactogenesis may be delayed

*Based on data from Riordan, J., & Auerbach, K. J. (1999). *Breastfeeding and human lactation* (2nd ed., pp. 163–220). Boston: Jones & Bartlett. Briggs, G. G., Freeman, R. K., & Yaffe, S. J. (1998). *Drugs in pregnancy and lactation* (5th ed.). Baltimore: Williams & Wilkins. Committee on Drugs, American Academy of Pediatrics. (1994). The transfer of drugs and other chemicals into human milk. *Pediatrics,* 93, 137–150. Taeusch, H., & Ballard, R. A. (1998). *Avery's diseases of the newborn* (7th ed., pp. 1348–1352). Philadelphia: Saunders.

Antihistamines

Diphenhydramine (Benadryl), pheniramine (Dimetane), Claritin, Allegra: May cause decreased milk supply; infant may become drowsy or irritable

Antimetabolites

Unknown, probably long-term anti-DNA effect on the infant; potentially very toxic

Antimicrobials

Aminoglycosides: May cause ototoxicity or nephrotoxicity if given for more than 2 weeks

Ampicillin: Skin rash, candidiasis; diarrhea

Chloramphenicol: Possible bone marrow suppression; too low a dose for Gray syndrome; refusal of breast

Methacycline: Possible inhibition of bone growth; may cause discoloration of the teeth; use should be avoided

Metronidazole (Flagyl): Possible neurologic disorders or blood dyscrasias; delay breastfeeding for 12 hours after dose

Penicillin: Possible allergic response; candidiasis

Quinolones (synthetic antibiotics): Can cause arthropathies

Sulfonamides: May cause hyperbilirubinemia; use contraindicated until infant over 1 week old

Tetracycline: Long-term use and large doses should be avoided; may cause tooth staining or inhibition of bone growth

Antithyroids

Thiouracil: Contraindicated during lactation; may cause goiter or agranulocytosis

Barbiturates

Propylthiouracil: Safe; monitor infant thyroid function
Phenothiazines: May produce sedation

Bronchodilators

Aminophylline: May cause insomnia or irritability in the infant
Ephedrine, cromolyn (Intal): Relatively safe

Caffeine

Excessive consumption may cause jitteriness or wakefulness

Cardiovascular

Methyldopa: Increase in milk volume

Propranolol (Inderal): May cause hypoglycemia; possibility of other blocking effects, especially if infant has renal or liver dysfunction

Quinidine: May cause arrhythmias in infant

Reserpine (Serpasil): Nasal stuffiness, lethargy, or diarrhea in infant

Corticosteroids

Adrenal suppression may occur with long-term administration of doses greater than 10 mg/day

Diuretics

Furosemide (Lasix): Not excreted in breast milk

Thiazide diuretics (Esidrix, Hydrodiuril, Oretic): Safe but can cause dehydration, reduce milk production

Heavy metals

Gold: Potentially toxic; gold salts—compatible with nursing
Mercury: Excreted in the milk and hazardous to infant

Hormones

Androgens: Suppress lactation
Thyroid hormones: May mask hypothyroidism

Laxatives

Peri-Colaces Ducolax: Relatively safe

Milk of magnesia, metamucil: Relatively safe

Narcotic analgesics

Codeine: Accumulation may lead to neonatal depression

Meperidine: May lead to neonatal depression

Morphine: Long-term use may cause newborn addiction

Nonnarcotic analgesics, NSAIDs

Acetaminophen (Tylenol): Relatively safe for short-term analgesia

Ibuprofen (Motrin): Safe

Propoxyphene (Darvon): May cause sleepiness and poor nursing in infant

Salicylates (aspirin): Safe after first week of life; monitor protime

Oral contraceptives

Combined estrogen/progestin pills: Significantly decrease milk supply; may alter milk composition; may cause gynecomastia in male infants

Progestin only (DMPA, Norplant): Safe if started after lactation is established

Radioactive materials for testing

Gallium citrate (^{67}G): Insignificant amount excreted in breast milk; no nursing for 2 weeks

Iodine: Contraindicated; may affect infant's thyroid gland

^{125}I: Discontinue nursing for 48 hours

^{131}I: Nursing should be discontinued until excretion is no longer significant; nursing may be resumed after 10 days

Technetium-99m: Discontinue nursing for 3 days (half-life = 6 hours)

Sedatives/tranquilizers

Diazepam (Valium): May accumulate to high levels; may increase neonatal jaundice; may cause lethargy and weight loss

Lithium: Contraindicated; may cause neonatal flaccidity and hypotonia

Substance abuse

Alcohol: Potential motor developmental delay; mild sedative effect

Amphetamines: Controversial; may cause irritability, poor sleeping pattern

Cocaine, crack: Extreme irritability, tachycardia, vomiting, apnea

Marijuana: Drowsiness

Heroin: Tremors, restlessness, vomiting, poor feeding

Nicotine (smoking): Shock, vomiting, diarrhea, decreased milk production

Appendix E
Selected Maternal Laboratory Values

Normal Maternal Laboratory Values

Test	Nonpregnant Values	Pregnant Values
Hematocrit	37%–47%	32%–42%
Hemoglobin	12–16 g/dL*	10–14 g/dL*
Platelets	150,000–350,000/mm^3	Significant increase 3 to 5 days after birth (predisposes to thrombosis)
Partial thrombo-plastin time (PTT)	12–14 seconds	Slight decrease in pregnancy and again in labor (placental site clotting)
Fibrinogen	250 mg/dL	400 mg/dL
Serum glucose:		
Fasting	70–80 mg/dL	65 mg/dL
2-hour postprandial	60–110 mg/dL	< 140 mg/dL
Total protein	6.7–8.3 g/dL	5.5–7.5 g/dL
White blood cell total	4500–10,000/mm^3	5000–15,000/mm^3
Polymorphonuclear cells	54%–62%	60%–85%
Lymphocytes	38%–46%	15%–40%

*At sea level.

Appendix F

Selected Newborn Laboratory Values

Normal Neonatal Laboratory Values

Test	Normal Values
Hematocrit	51%–56%
Hemoglobin	16.5 g/dL (cord blood)
Platelets	150,000–400,000/mm^3
White blood cell total	18,000/mm^3
White blood cell differential:	
Bands	1600/mm^3 (9%)
Polymorphonuclear (segs)	9400/mm^3 (52%)
Eosinophils	400/mm^3 (2.2%)
Basophils	100/mm^3 (0.6%)
Lymphocytes	5500/mm^3 (31%)
Monocytes	1050/mm^3 (5.8%)
Serum glucose	40–80 mg/dL
Serum electrolytes:	
Sodium	135–147 mEq/L
Potassium	4–6 mEq/L
Chloride	90–114 mEq/L
Carbon dioxide	15–25 mEq/L
Bicarbonate	18–23 mEq/L
Calcium	7–10 mg/dL

*At sea level.

Appendix G

Spanish Translations of English Phrases[1]

This appendix includes phrases you might find helpful in working with families during pregnancy, labor and birth, and after the birth. There are many ways to phrase questions. We have chosen some statements we consider essential and have tried to phrase them in a straightforward way. The phrases are designed to help you in situations in which translation is not possible at the moment.

This list begins with introductory statements, which are presented in a logical conversational flow. The remaining phrases are arranged according to the phases of pregnancy and birth during which they are most applicable.

Essential Introductory Phrases	**Frases Introductoras Esenciales**
Hello.	Hola.
I am a nurse.	Soy enfermera (enfermero).[2]
I am a student nurse.	Soy estudiante de enfermería.
My name is _____	Mi nombre es _____ Me llamo _____
What is your name?	¿Cuál es su nombre? ¿Cómo se llama?

---

1. Prepared by Elizabeth Medina, PhD, Associate Professor of Spanish, Regis University, Denver, Colorado.
2. In Spanish, nouns that end in *a* indicate female gender. Nouns that end in *o* indicate male gender.

What name should I call you?	¿Cómo quiere que la llamemos?
	¿Cómo quiere ser llamada?
Thank you.	Gracias.
Please.	Por favor.
Is someone here with you?	¿Hay alquien aquí con usted?
Does he (she) speak English?	¿Habla él (ella) English?
Goodbye.	Adiós.

Phrases for the Antepartal Period

Frases para el Periodo Prenatal

Are you taking any medications now?	¿Está tomando algunas medicinas ahora?
Show me the medicine bottles, please.	Por favor, muéstreme los frascos.
Have you ever had trouble with your blood pressure?	¿Ha tenido problemas alguna vez con la presión arterial?
When was the first day of your last period?	¿Cuál fue el primer día de su última regla?
	¿Cuál fue el primer día de su última menstruación?
Have you had any spotting or bleeding since your last period?	¿Ha sangrado o ha tenido manchas de sangre desde su última regla?
Have you been on birth control pills?	¿Ha estado tomando píldoras anticonceptivas?
When did you stop taking them?	¿Cuándo dejó de tomarlas?
Do you have an intrauterine device (IUD)?	¿Usa un aparato intrauterino?
How many times have you been pregnant?	¿Cuántas veces ha estado usted embarazada?
Are you having any problems with your pregnancy?	¿Tiene problemas con su embarazo?

Is there anything worrying you?	¿Hay algo o alguna cosa que la preocupe?
I would like to take your blood pressure.	Quisiera tomarle la presión arterial.
I would like to take your pulse.	Quisiera tomarle el pulso.
I would like to take your temperature.	Quisiera tomarle la temperatura.
I would like to listen to your heart and lungs.	Quisiera escucharle el corazon y los pulmones.
I would like to check your uterus.	Quisiera examinarle el útero.
Would you please urinate in this cup and leave it in the bathroom?	¿Puede orinar en este vaso y dejarlo en el baño?
Please stand up.	Por favor, levántese.
Please sit down.	Por favor, siéntese.
Please lie down.	Por favor, acuéstese.

Phrases Related to Client Safety

Frases Relacionadas con la Seguridad del Cliente

I would like to talk to you alone.	Quisiera hablar a solas con usted.
Are you safe at home?	¿Sufre de peligros en casa?
Are you afraid of your partner?	¿Le tiene miedo a su compañero?
During your pregnancy has your partner hit, slapped, kicked, or punched you?	Durante su embarazo, ¿la ha golpeado? ¿la ha abofeteado? ¿la ha pateado? o ¿le ha dado puñetazos?
How many times?	¿Cuántas veces?
Do you have someone for support?	¿Cuénta con alguien que la pueda ayudar?

Questions the Mother or Father May Ask

How big is my baby?

How much does the baby weigh now?

When will I feel my baby move?

Phrases for the Intrapartal Period

Note: Review the Essential Introductory Phrases for beginning conversation.

Are you having labor pains?

Are you having contractions?

Are you having pain?

Do you need medicine for pain?

Do you need to urinate?

This is a bedpan to urinate in.

Can I help you to the bathroom?

Do you need to have a bowel movement?

Has your bag of water broken?

Have you had any bright-red bleeding during your pregnancy?

How many births have you had?

I need to do a vaginal examination.

Posibles Preguntas que Madres y Padres Hacen

¿De qué tamaño es el (la) bebé ahora?

¿Cuánto pesa el bebé ahora?

¿Cuándo lo (la) voy a sentir moverse?

Frases Durante el Parto

Nota: Repase las frases introductoras para comenzar una conversación.

¿Tiene dolores de parto?

¿Tiene contracciones?

¿Tiene dolores?

¿Necesita medicina para el dolor?

¿Necesita orinar?

Aquí tiene el bacín (la chata) (el pato) para orinar.

¿La ayudo a ir al baño?

¿Necesita mover el vientre (obrar)? Necesita "hacer caca"—coloquial

¿Se le ha roto la bolsa de aqua(s)?

¿Ha tenido algún sangramiento de color rojo durante su embarazo?

¿Cuántos niños le han nacido?

Necesito hacerle un examen vaginal.

I will help you.	La voy a ayudar.
I will stay with you.	Me quedaré con usted.
Please pant. I will show you how.	Por favor, jadee. Le voy a mostrar cómo.
Please do not push.	No puje ahora.
Push now.	Puje ahora.
Stop pushing.	Pare de pujar. No puje más.
The doctor needs to do a cesarean birth.	El doctor le va a hacer una operación cesárea.
This is medicine for your pain. You will feel better soon.	Esta medicina es para el dolor. Va a sentirse mejor pronto.
When is your baby supposed to be born?	¿Cuándo está supuesto a nacer el bebé?

January	February	enero	febrero
March	April	marzo	abril
May	June	mayo	junio
July	August	julio	agosto
September	October	septiembre	octubre
November	December	noviembre	diciembre

What is your doctor's name?	¿Cuál es el nombre de su doctor?
What is your midwife's name?	¿Cuál es el nombre de su comadrona (partera)?
Your baby is having a little trouble now.	El bebé está pasando por algunos problemas. El bebé está sufriendo algunas dificultades.
I need to put this oxygen mask on you. It will help your baby. It may smell funny, but it is OK.	Le voy a poner esta máscara de oxígeno. Va a ayudar al bebé. Huele extraño, pero no hay problemas.
Please turn on your left side.	Por favor voltéese al lado izquierdo.

Please turn on your right side.

Por favor voltéese al lado derecho.

Your baby is OK.

El bebé está bien.

Phrases for the Postpartal Period and the Newborn Area

Frases para el Periodo Despues del Parto y el Area del Recien Nacido

Note: Review the Essential Introductory Phrases for beginning conversation.

Nota: Repase las frases introductoras para comenzar una conversación.

Are you hungry?

¿Tiene hambre?

Are you thirsty?

¿Tiene sed?

Are you cold?

¿Tiene frío?

Are you tired?

¿Está cansada?

I am going to put antibiotic ointment in the baby's eyes. It will help protect your baby from some infections.

Le voy a poner al bebé un ungüento antibiótico alrededor de los ojos. Lo (la) va a proteger contra infecciones.

I am going to take some blood from your baby's foot to check the blood sugar and hematocrit.

Le voy a sacar sangre del pie al bebé para determinar el azúcar de la sangre y el hematocrítico.

If your baby begins to spit up, please turn him (her) on his (her) side.

Si el bebé comienza a vomitar, colóquelo (colóquela) de costado.

It may help to position your baby like this.

Lo (la) ayudará—si lo coloca así.

Lo (la) ayudaría—si lo colocara así.

I would like to suggest that you clean your nipples this way before you breastfeed your baby.

Es bueno que se lave los pezones de esta manera antes de darle el pecho al bebé.

I would like to suggest that you clean your baby's cord this way.

Es mejor para el bebé que le lave el ombligo de esta manera.

I would like to suggest that you bathe your baby this way.	Es mejor que lo (la) bañe de esta manera.
I would like to suggest that you clean your baby's penis this way.	Es mejor que le limpie el pene así.
I would like you to fold the diaper this way.	Le sugiero que doble el pañal así.
I would like to suggest that you fasten the diaper this way.	Le sugiero que asegure el pañal así.
I would like to suggest that you take the baby's temperature this way.	Tómele la temperatura así.
I need to check your breasts, your uterus, your flow, your stitches, your legs and feet.	Necesito examinarle los pechos, el útero, el flujo, los puntos, las piernas y los pies.
I need to feel your uterus.	Necesito examinarle el útero.
I need to massage your uterus.	Necesito darle un masaje en la región del útero.
Place your baby on its side.	Coloque al bebé de costado.
Place the baby's used diaper here.	Coloque aquí los pañales usados.
Please rub your uterus every half hour to keep it firm. I will show you how.	Necesita darse un masaje en la región del útero cada media hora para mantenerlo firme. Le voy a mostrar cómo.
Would you like to see your baby now?	¿Quiere ver a su bebé ahora?
Would you like me to help you feed your baby?	¿Quiere que le ayude a alimentarlo (la)?
Your baby needs a car seat to go home in.	El (la) bebé necesita un asiento para bebés en el automóvil.

Special Neonatal Needs

We are giving your baby oxygen.

Your baby is having some problems breathing.

Your baby needs extra help.

Your baby needs to go to a special care nursery.

Necesidades del Recien Nacido

Le vamos a dar oxígeno al (a la) bebé.

El (la) bebé tiene problemas al respirar.

El (la) bebé necesita ayuda especial.

El (la) bebé necesita ir a la sala de cuidados especiales para bebés

Appendix H

Guidelines for Working with a Deaf Client and an Interpreter[1]

1. First, remember that it requires trust on the part of the client to allow nonsigning caregivers and an interpreter into his or her life.

2. It is important to use a registered interpreter. Medical interpreters are registered with the Registry of Interpreters for the Deaf. Although family members and friends may offer to interpret, it is best to use registered medical interpreters because they are bound to translate the client's and nurse's words accurately without adding any other opinion.

3. Greet the client and family with a handshake and a body posture that indicates welcome. You may point to your name tag and use the American Sign Language (ASL) alphabet cards to spell out your name. The client may wish to select cards to indicate his or her name. Rapport will be especially important as you work together, and making the effort to provide a greeting as you would with speaking clients will help establish rapport.

4. Once the interpreter is present, continue to look at the client and speak directly to her or him. There will be a temptation to look at the interpreter, and it will help to remember that you are speaking to the client.

1. Prepared with the kind assistance of Mr. Gerald Dement, Interpreter Coordinator, Pikes Peak Center on Deafness, Colorado Springs, Colorado.

5. Avoid phrasing your words as if you are talking to the interpreter. For example, "Can you tell her . . ." Instead, phrase your questions as you do with hearing clients. For example, "I am going to ask you some questions now."

6. Depend on the deaf client to ask questions.

7. Look at the client's face for signs of difficulty in understanding. Deaf clients have a behavior of "gesturing" which involves shaking their head as if to indicate "yes" even when they do not understand. If the client is nodding "yes," ask her or him to repeat the directions you have just given.

8. Be as direct as possible. Keep to what you want to know or what you want to convey. Speak in short sentences using nontechnical words. Avoid colloquial or slang words. Be sure to explain what you want to do, before you do it. For instance, tell her you want to start an IV and explain the equipment. Then, with her permission, start the IV.

9. Be aware that deaf clients may have difficulty understanding when to take medications. It will be helpful to associate taking medications or completing some treatment/activity with meals. (For instance, while showing her the two capsules she is to take when she goes home, tell her to take the two capsules at breakfast and another two capsules at bedtime). Avoid saying, "Take two capsules at 8 A.M., 2 P.M., and 12 A.M."

10. The difference in interpreting time may also affect obtaining a history. It is best to begin with a specific event in the past and work forward.

What to Do until the Interpreter Arrives

1. Role play as much as possible.

2. Demonstrate what you want the client to do or what you want to do.

3. Be resourceful.

4. Remember that some deaf clients can read lips. Some may read written language, but use care in assuming the client understands.

What to Do to Prepare for Working with a Deaf Client

1. Contact local agencies that work with deaf clients to see what resources are available. Ask about classes in ASL. Learning some basic signs will be very helpful until an interpreter arrives.

2. Read to learn more about the deaf culture. Contact your local agency or the National Information Center on Deafness, Silver Spring, Maryland, for suggestions on books you might read.

3. Investigate your health facility. What is available to assist you? Look at any videos used for teaching in the maternal-child unit and note if they have captions. Remember that many deaf clients do not read written language, so it will be important to review the content on the video with an interpreter present.

Sign Language for Health Care Professionals

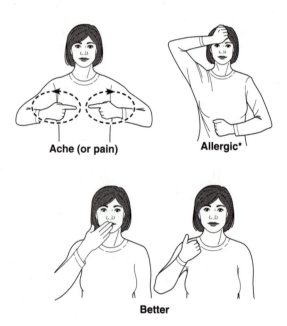

Ache (or pain)

Allergic*

Better

*Indicates signs that are in manually signed English. Those without an asterisk are in American Sign Language.

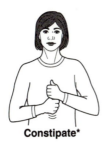

Constipate*

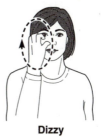

Dizzy

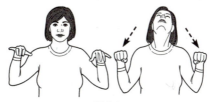

Faint

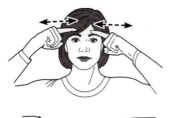

Headache

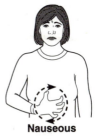

Nauseous

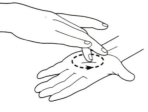

Medicine

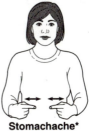

Stomachache*

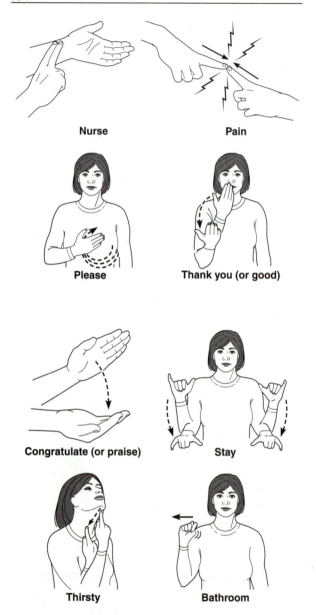

Nurse

Pain

Please

Thank you (or good)

Congratulate (or praise)

Stay

Thirsty

Bathroom

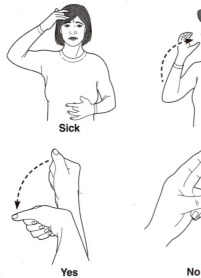

Sick

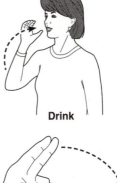

Drink

Yes

No

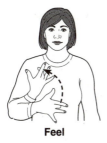

Feel

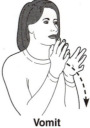

Vomit

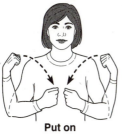

Put on

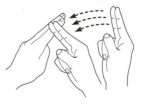

Name

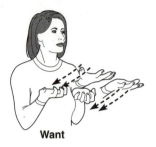

Want

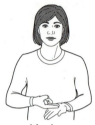

Lie down

Index